MW01125711

Trigeminal
Neuralgia
Without
Drugs

Alex Guerrero

ISBN: 9798373140577

Dedication

I dedicate this book to all the people affected by a chronic disease and non-conformists from the point of view of allopathic medicine, to all my followers and to all those who trusted me during my trajectory in Natural Medicines.

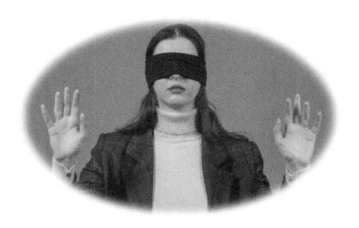

Remove the blindfold of your deepest beliefs to overcome your disease.

Alex Guerrero

Notes

All the methods explained in this volume are complementary therapies, they NEVER replace a diagnosis, a medical, pharmacological or surgical treatment. In case of emergency, you should ALWAYS call emergency services. The supervision of a qualified physician is recommended, and at no time should the treatment be discontinued without the physician's consent.

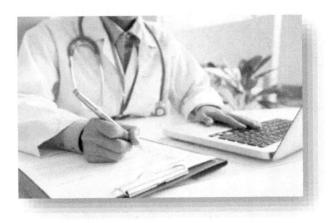

With this book, I only intend to show you the path that led me to healing through my experience of natural therapies. I have done my best to write this book in the simplest and most didactic language possible in order to make it accessible to all audiences and avoiding the use of difficult technical terms. All texts and images, with the exception of royalty-free images, are the property of Alex Guerrero and may not be copied or reproduced without his express permission.

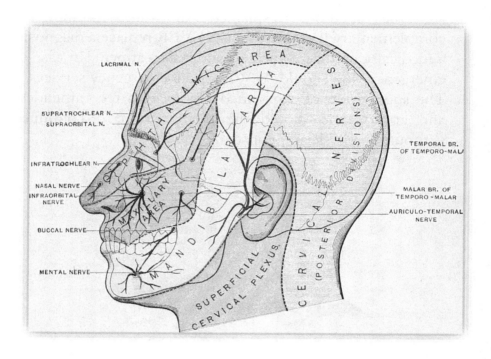

Introduction

If you have come across this book, you have probably been suffering from this terrible condition for some time without having received much information about it. You have probably consulted several neurologists who have given you only limited chemical relief of symptoms, but who have left you in a state of permanent physical and mental exhaustion. You will have realized that the medication(s) you take every day are only hiding something more serious that refuses to let you live in peace. You may have asked yourself dozens of times: why did this terrible thing happen to me? I'm sure you live in constant fear waiting for the next electric shock, begging your body not to punish you too much this time. You may have waited so long for your illness to end that you no longer even dream of this day of atonement. You've probably spent hours searching the web and consulting Mr. GOOGLE, desperately looking for something more, a clearer answer or a last resort remedy. You will have read so much information that I wouldn't be surprised if, in addition to leaving you even more uninformed, you were even more tormented. If your specialist suggested surgery, he or she may have given you some hope, but at the same time, you may have been frightened by the low success rate and high level of risk. If they suggested that you might receive gamma radiation treatment, you may have been alarmed by the high price tag for such a low success rate, or frightened by the high level of radiation toxicity to your body for the rest of your life. Perhaps you've been offered a surgery that would render your face numb forever, and you're past the point of weighing the pros and cons, only to do it as a last resort. Or worse, you may be considering ending your pain in the most radical way possible, by cutting short your life to overcome the most terrible pain a human being can endure.

You probably already know that Trigeminal Neuralgia is considered the worst pain known to man. A pain so terrible, that medical science often finds no remedy. How, in the century of the most remarkable inventions and the gigantic progress of mankind, did we not manage to make this dreadful disease disappear? A pathology such as trigeminal neuralgia remains a notable failure for conventional medicine. It is one more hindrance, like cancer or the more than 7000 other rare diseases listed by the World Health Organization. I am not going to comment again on what is going on in the management of diseases in medicine and pharmaceuticals, as I have already amply demonstrated in my previous books, "How I defeated Trigeminal Neuralgia" and "The Occult Truth of Hypertension".

In this work, I wanted to get to the heart of the matter and focus directly on the relief and disappearance of your condition. I wanted to open a door to hope and show you that this disease has a solution beyond chemical drugs or any surgery. Not only have I suffered from Trigeminal Neuralgia for 25 years, but, like you, I have been an inveterate researcher for this quarter of a century, on the trail of truth, in search of the definitive natural solution.

After 25 years of research, trial and error, I am very proud to have found the ultimate solution. A method that has worked for me and for all the Trigeminal Neuralgia sufferers who have tried it. No matter what label was given to your neuralgia (atypical, idiopathic, postherpetic, pressure on the nerve by a blood vessel, trauma...), you will find here the answers to all your doubts, and the definitive remedy that will give you back the life you lost at some point in your life. When you reach the last page of this book, you will have the maximum amount of information to defeat your greatest enemy and find peace. But you will not only remove this adversary that lives inside you, you will also improve a myriad of aspects of your overall health, both physically and emotionally. In this volume, I offer 19 natural treatments to combat trigeminal neuralgia. The first three are the result of a quarter century of scientific research, the results of which will surprise you. I have added 3 additional treatments that work on the emotions and 13 additional or optional therapies that you can choose to speed up the healing process. This book will be a battery of weapons of mass destruction for you that will annihilate your worst enemy and you will be able, under your doctor's supervision, to abandon medication and regain the reins of the precious life you once had. This book is an improved and expanded version of my previous work on neuralgia. I have added to my first work themes that I discovered later. It has become the only existing book of this caliber to date. The Definitive Naturopathic Guide to Trigeminal Neuralgia.

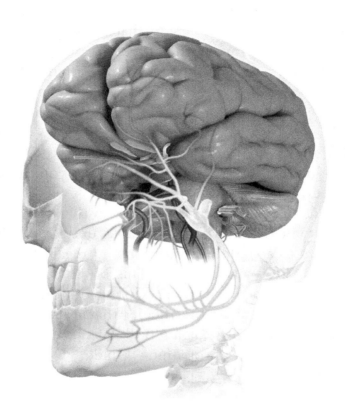

"Official" definition

Trigeminal neuralgia is also known as suicidal disease or Fothergill's disease (who discovered it clinically in 1776).

It is a neuropathic condition of the cranial nerve V that causes episodes of electric shock-like seizures on the side of the face, in the eyes, mouth, paranasal cavities, scalp, cheeks, forehead and jaw. The fact that it is called a suicidal disease has nothing to do with the fact that it necessarily leads to the end of one's life, but with the unbearable character of the pain generated by this disease. The trigeminal nerve has 3 specific branches: the ophthalmic nerve, the maxillary nerve and the mandibular nerve. The disease can occur in one, two or all three branches.

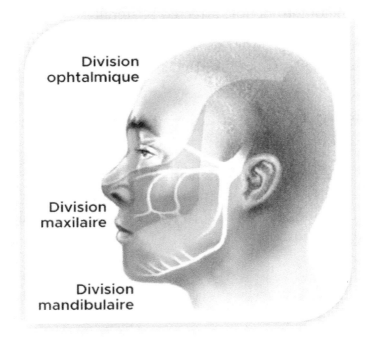

In isolation, the impact is as follows:

- The 1st branch (ophthalmic) represents 2% of cases.
- The 2nd branch (maxillary) represents 20% of cases.
- The 3rd branch (mandibular) accounts for 17% of cases.

As a group, the impact is as follows:

- The 1st and 2nd branches together account for 14% of cases.
- The 2nd and 3rd branches together account for 42% of cases.
- The 3 branches together account for 5% of cases.

There is a greater number of people affected on the right cheek with 60% of the cases, the left cheek represents 39%, and 1% belong to people affected bilaterally.

The disease usually appears from the age of 50, but this is not always the case and it affects women more often than men.

The annual incidence is estimated at 3-4 persons per 100,000 population.

One of the major problems with this condition is that it is still relatively unknown to many general practitioners and is not well diagnosed. Referral to a neurological specialization is of great importance.

The description of the pain is very similar to a high intensity electric shock, which can last from a fraction of a second to several minutes and the episodes can last from a few minutes to several months at a time, and then may suddenly subside and return after a while.

It is often triggered by a stimulus on the affected side of the face, which may be a draught, eating, brushing teeth, talking, or even a simple smile or emotion.

.

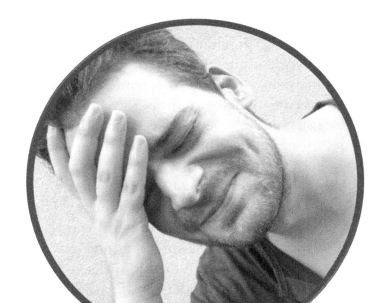

Danger, drugs in sight.

It has already been proven many times that chemotherapy is very ineffective and in many cases even makes the problem worse. Both oncologists and pharmaceutical companies have always lied about this and hidden its ineffectiveness from patients. Recent scientific studies show that some of the most commonly used drugs, such as Taxol or Adriamycin, can cause metastasis, mitochondrial dysfunction, fatigue, weakness, oxidative stress and loss of muscle mass. These are just a few brief examples.

As Dr. Enric Costa Vercher said in 2019 in a significant and rigorous work after 25 years of data collection and exhaustive analysis: scientific medicine has become an industrial medicine unable to properly care for the sick. This doctor blames the medical system and its drugs for many rare diseases, autoimmune disorders and even infertility.

But what fascinated me the most was his assertion, which I was able to verify several times: the course "History of Medicine" is not taught during the medical career although it is on the curriculum, and the subject is given as a pass. In other words, this subject is devalued in order to make them work doctors. Now, I also understand how few hours are taught in nutrition, when it is the very basis of health.

Dr. Costa recognizes that it is important to the industry that physicians know nothing about the history of their medical ancestors so they can manipulate them. And they are educated as if they were the first doctors in history, preventing another view of medicine. Is it because two hundred years ago medicine was very close to alternative and natural medicine that they are undermining? Or is it because there is no interest in shedding light on the Rockefeller story? I have no doubt about that.

My own doctor friends have told me, "We are not doctors, we are drug administrators. And we already know that drugs don't cure, so what are doctors for, to fatten the accounts of pharmaceutical companies?

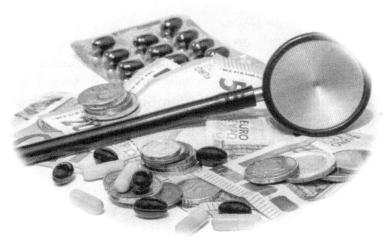

It is more than proven that a lie repeated endlessly in the media becomes an absolute truth. One of these lies is that "medicine is progressing and has been able to eradicate many diseases".

So why are there more diseases than ever? Another lie is that "people are living better and longer", thanks to vaccines and antibiotics. If you have read "The Occult Truth of High Blood Pressure", you already know the answer about vaccines. As for antibiotics, studies show that they are already causing countless deaths by preventing the body from making its own antibodies and many doctors warn that in a few years they will become the leading cause of death. As for longevity, nothing has been proven.

In the 19th century, the microscope was invented and microbes were discovered. They found that they were everywhere. This observation led doctors to position themselves in two very distinct groups. The first group, composed of the vast majority of physicians and biologists, including several Nobel Prize winners, was inclined to affirm that these microbes could not be bad for the organism and that they even helped us in certain functions, as was later demonstrated.

As for the second group, the thinking was quite the opposite. These scientists thought that these microbes were harmful to us and brought all kinds of diseases. This second group was led by the famous Louis Pasteur, who was not a doctor (which people often ignore).

Pasteur was in the wine and spirits industry.

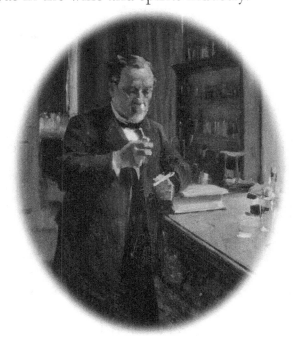

Louis Pasteur

This small group won over the chemical industry with the financial support of the alcohol merchant and imposed the famous "infection theory". It has been taught in medical schools to this day and is taken for granted by most doctors who constantly prescribe antibiotics and antiseptics. Often, the major diseases are viral and cannot be destroyed by antibiotics. But I still know doctors who prescribe such drugs to attack a flu. What happens with that? That the body receiving antibiotics is weakened and will contract the next cold or flu more virulently. People already take antibiotics too easily for a sore throat without knowing whether it is bacterial or viral. If they could figure out what is really happening in their body after taking the drug, I doubt they would.

They have succeeded in making people feel privileged to have access to a modern health care system when they don't know that they are real laboratory guinea pigs on whom all sorts of products and substances are tested with impunity. These do not frighten us because we are told that they have passed health checks. So why are countless drugs withdrawn every year that have caused damage, sometimes irreparable? Haven't they also passed these exhaustive controls? In Spain alone, the Ministry of Health withdraws every year more than a thousand drugs from the market (some probably because of commercial problems, but many others because they are dangerous). To cite just one case, Valsartan, the high blood pressure drug that was withdrawn from the market because it contained impurities that were probably carcinogenic, highlighted a fact: as in the automotive, technology and textile sectors, large Asian countries are cheap manufacturers that companies turn to. According to sources close to generic drug makers, "it is normal for companies to turn to raw material suppliers located in China or India, as about 80% of certified manufacturers are located there, and those in other parts of the world do not have the capacity or availability to supply the entire pharmaceutical industry. Do these Eastern laboratories have the same, supposedly rigorous, controls as in Europe or America? The difference with natural medicine is that the substances used have been known for thousands of years, whereas the effects of industrial pharmaceuticals are not known in the long term. This is why many doctors are already attributing new diseases to these new chemicals.

People are not aware that every time they take a pill, there is a positive or negative effect. It's like a roulette wheel, you never know what you're really doing to your body. I think the real problem is often impatience. I mean, people take an aspirin or a Nolotil or a Paracetamol at the drop of a hat. Nobody wants to wait for it to pass naturally or take an herbal remedy. These people are unaware that their liver is becoming more and more toxic and that if this organ is not functioning properly, the rest of the body will not function any better. Just think that the liver has over 2,000 chemical functions.

It has been recorded that in Spain alone, in 2020, some 22,400,000 units of Nolotil (analgesic), 16,600,000 of Adiro (aspirin), 15,900,000 of Paracetamol were sold. It is enough to mention the first three to get an idea of what is going on. If we study medicines in depth, which nobody does, we will discover that there are scientific research results that clearly show that many of these products that claim to save our lives have very dangerous contraindications and, even worse, that they are passed over in silence.

Thus, we can say that medicine is often nothing more than a belief system whose contrary opinion will be crushed by the media.

Another major medical obstacle is that most doctors believe that if one drug works, two will work even better. So when after a while your liver is saturated and your neuralgia gets worse again, your doctor will combine anticonvulsants with painkillers. Doctors take it for granted that a second drug with a different action can act in a complementary way. In this way, we increase the risk of side effects and multiply liver toxicity.

The neurologist has most likely prescribed a drug or combination of drugs to relieve physical suffering. I have found in many cases that medications do not always work as well as expected. In addition to not addressing the root of the problem, i.e., the primary cause, they only mask the symptoms, and very often do not even accomplish this goal, leading the patient to a state of anxiety, fear and despair. Sometimes these medications only work for a while while the body gets used to them. In other cases, they lead the patient to an overdose, to a state close to drug addiction and to the near nullity of a normal life.

At other times, the combination of three or four drugs only allows for an apparently normal life with the negative consequences of an intoxicated body and altered mental state.

These formulations are often anticonvulsants such as those taken by epileptics.

There are many anticonvulsants, most of which tend to reduce the electrochemical activity of the brain by interacting with neurotransmitter receptors such as GABA and glutamate; others block sodium and calcium channels, thereby controlling voltage, and some of the mechanisms of action remain unknown at this time.

The most common are oxcarbazepine, carbamazepine, clonazepam, phenytoin, lamotrigine, gabapentin, baclofen, etc.

Of these, oxcarbazepine and gabapentin tend to be the most "effective" overall.

I will describe their possible counterproductive impacts as an example...

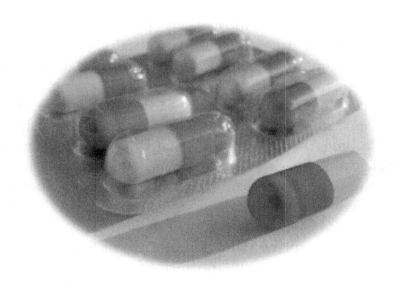

Oxcarbazepine

Common and very common side effects are generally as follows

- Fatigue
- Headache
- Dizziness
- Drowsiness
- Feeling dizzy (nausea or lightheaded)
- Double or blurred vision
- Low sodium levels in the blood
- Trembling
- Coordination problems
- Involuntary eye movements
- Feelings of anxiety and nervousness
- Feelings of depression
- Mood swings
- Skin rash
- Weakness
- Memory problems
- Difficulty concentrating
- Apathy
- Agitation
- Confusion
- Constipation or diarrhea
- Stomach pain (abdominal)
- Acne
- Hair loss

Gabapentine

Common and very common side effects are generally:

- Viral infection
- Feeling of drowsiness
- Dizziness and incoordination
- Feeling tired
- Fever
- Pneumonia or respiratory infection
- Urinary tract infection
- Inflammation of the ear
- Low white blood cell count
- Anorexia or increased appetite
- Anger towards others
-Confusion, mood swings, depression, anxiety, nervousness, thought disorders
- Seizures or tremors
- Difficulty speaking
- Loss of memory
- Trembling
- Difficulty sleeping
- Headaches
- Skin sensitivity or decreased sensation
- Unusual eye movements
- Increased, decreased or absent reflexes
- Blurred vision, double vision
- Dizziness
- Increased blood pressure, redness or dilation of blood vessels
- Difficulty breathing, bronchitis, sore throat, cough, dry nose
- Vomiting (dizziness), nausea (feeling lightheaded)

- Tooth problems, swollen gums
- Diarrhea, upset stomach, indigestion, constipation, dry mouth or throat, flatulence
- Facial swelling, bruising, rashes, itching, acne.
- Joint pain, muscle pain, back pain, spasms
- Incontinence
- Erection difficulties
- Swelling of the legs and arms or swelling that may affect the face, trunk and extremities, difficulty walking, weakness, pain, aches and pains, flu-like symptoms
- weight gain
- Accidental injuries, fractures, scrapes and abrasions..

And that's not to mention the dangers during pregnancy, breastfeeding, in children, and the less frequent or rare effects.

Yes, dear reader, the list is exorbitant and grim. We often don't stop to look at the package insert. If we do, we may find that the drugs are not as "virtuous" as we think. All of these side effects translate into new conditions in the long run that will require new antidotes, or our bodies will simply go into a state of collapse due to the high toxicity, facilitating the creation of new disorders or the worsening of the ones we already have. In the case of this pathology, medication will be prescribed for life and, hopefully, with annual tests to assess the damage.

The cause remains a big question mark for medicine.

As mentioned above, the diagnosis is not always easy, and it is often confused with toothache, migraine or other types of facial neuralgia that have nothing to do with the type or intensity.

Medicine has found a link with multiple sclerosis because this disease affects the myelin of the nerves (the insulating layer that surrounds them). This layer, or sheath, made up of proteins and fatty substances, allows electrical impulses to travel quickly and efficiently along the neurons. If this layer is damaged, it can cause deep pain.

Another possible cause, according to allopathic medicine, is a tumor that compresses the trigeminal nerve.

Accidental injuries, brain abnormalities, surgical injuries, facial trauma or strokes should also not be ruled out. Often, doctors tell us that it is simply due to a blood vessel compressing the nerve at the beginning of its course, and affecting its myelin again. But I have to say that most often the diagnosis is idiopathic, which means nothing more than a spontaneous manifestation or an unknown cause. This word sounds better than writing "I don't know" on a medical report.

But is it really so?

The Real Culprit of Trigeminal Neuralgia.

In reality, and this is the reason why medicine is unable to cure this terrible pathology, is that the only real cause of trigeminal neuralgia is the **HERPES ZOSTER VIRUS**.

It can be classified as atypical, idiopathic, postherpetic, cavitary alveolar osteopathy or due to a supposed vein that mistakenly presses on the nerve. But the only real cause is viral, which means that they are all actually postherpetic. People with multiple sclerosis share the same virus, which is why it coincides with T.N. And you might ask me why traditional medicine hasn't discovered this? Well, I can tell you that it has been discovered, outside of conventional medicine, but for some reason there is no point in publishing it. The same thing happened with multiple sclerosis or cancer. Many naturopaths have known for years that these are viral problems (of strains of the Epstein-Barr virus in particular, of the herpes family) and we were treating these problems antivirally correctly and successfully, but it was only in 2022 that conventional medical science publicly recognized this, while before that many were laughing at our corporation. Is it because of the commercial interests of the pharmaceutical companies? Is it because they refuse to admit that natural medicine is often more effective and more powerful? Is it because synthetic pharmacological antiviral drugs are not very effective? Is it because of the lack of training of physicians in nutrition? Is it because vaccines against these diseases are appearing out of nowhere? Will there be a vaccine for T.N. in the near future? Let everyone make their own conclusions. I think I have already given enough convincing data in my previous books.

And that is why they fail to solve the enigma and why doctors label the pathology, rightly or wrongly, and prescribe one or more drugs for life, without any improvement and, in most cases, worsening the symptoms with time, because the drugs do not cure but only temporarily camouflage the symptoms and intoxicate the body even more. This last fact aggravates the disease later on, whereas medicine attributes it to the fact that it is the pathology that naturally and falsely worsens with time.

The point is that ALL cases of trigeminal neuralgia are caused by the herpes zoster virus. One thing that should be clear to all doctors and patients is that the herpes zoster virus lives deep in the liver and does not always circulate in the blood, so blood tests are not able to determine with certainty whether you have such a viral load. Blood tests cannot detect the virus in any organ, only in the blood. We were able to verify that in all cases of neuralgia, the virus was present. This virus is usually contracted in childhood during varicella. It is exactly the same virus, even though it is one of the 30 existing varieties. When the child has passed the symptoms, it does not mean that the virus has simply left the body, but that the virus, attenuated, hides in its favorite place, in the depths of the liver (it can stay there for decades) where it will receive the pathogens it likes the most. These pathogens can be radiation, heavy metals, pesticides, hormones and all sorts of other crap that enters the body, whether through the mouth, nose or skin. Everything goes through the big processor called the liver.

If it gets the right pathogens to strengthen it, the virus will start releasing neurotoxins that travel up the phrenic or vagal nerve to the jaw and cause the famous electric shocks. The virus itself moves and settles in this part of the body, releasing waves of viral debris that damage the nerve. But it is not only reinforced by toxins, but also by a physical or emotional shock due to the cortisol or adrenaline released by the adrenal glands at that time. There are many cases of neuralgia after a blow to the jaw accidentally caused by the dentist or by a shock in another type of accident. This virus likes these hormones. Your task will be to protect your liver from this virus, keep away from toxins so as not to strengthen it and regulate your hormones, all in a natural way.

The herpes zoster virus not only releases dermotoxins, which we commonly know as shingles, but it can also release neurotoxins that impair nerves such as the 5th cranial nerve. We are talking about the same pathology with different impacts.

COMBINATIONS THAT CAUSE NEURALGIA

HERPES ZOSTER VIRUS + RADIATION

HERPES ZOSTER VIRUS + HEAVY METALS

HERPES ZOSTER VIRUS + DDT

HERPES ZOSTER VIRUS + CORTISOL OR ADRENALINE (MAY ALSO BE DUE TO PHYSICAL OR EMOTIONAL TRAUMA)

Radiation is everywhere, from cell phones to airplane flights to the X-rays and CT scans we get at the clinic. Heavy metals are also ubiquitous in our environment, from the air we breathe to the food we eat to dental amalgams. When I say DDT, it can be any pesticide, insecticide, fungicide...
Cortisol and adrenaline, two hormones that our body naturally produces when a stressful situation arises. Cortisol is also triggered by physical impact or emotional trauma, even in childhood.

What should we do then?

Eliminate the forbidden foods that we will see below. These foods strengthen the virus that attacks us without mercy. Our diet should be based on fruits and vegetables and completely avoid fats and oils, at least until we recover.

Of course, I don't expect you to become a vegetarian (I myself am not, although it has been proven to improve all health problems), but it should be 80% of your diet. You shouldn't just have chicken with vegetables, for example, you need vegetables with chicken. Vegetables and fruits should not be just a side dish but the key element of your health and the main course.

Take the utmost care of your liver, where the herpes zoster virus hides, which causes the neurotoxins that cause neuralgia.

Take the right supplements and foods to increase the liver's power to fight toxins and the virus (I'll give you a complete liver cleansing regimen that takes 10 days if you're interested).

Take foods and supplements that allow the chelation of heavy metals that we have in our body (I will give you a recipe for a wonderful shake.) and drink lots of water (not tap water) to allow them to leave the body.

Avoid exposure to electromagnetic radiation and DDT.

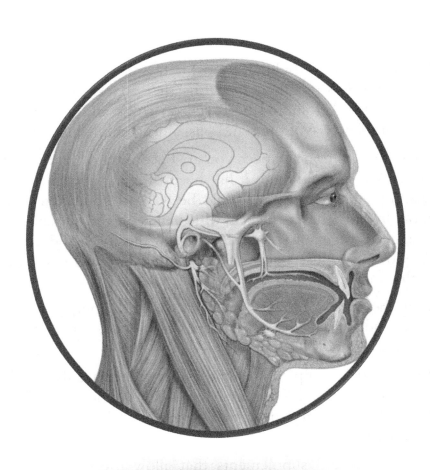

THREE-PHASE SYSTEM

Here is how this new treatment is structured. I have divided it into 3 major parts: THE 3 PHASES.

- **PHASE I: LIVER CLEANSING.** In this phase, we will focus on the elements that are detrimental to the health of the liver and the foods, herbs and supplements that will help this organ cleanse itself in the most optimal way possible. No other treatment to date is more effective than this. This phase can last from 10 to 30 days.

- **PHASE II: CHELATION.** This treatment must be done after the liver cleansing. This is when the liver is really strong and ready to eliminate the toxic heavy metals buried deep inside. We will see what these metals are and how they enter our body. Again, we will discuss the best chelating foods, herbs and supplements, and how to do it. This phase should last at least 30 days. I will also give you the recipe for the best heavy metal detox shake available today.

- **PHASE III: NATURAL SUPPLEMENTS FOR TRIGEMINAL NEURALGIA.** In this phase and after having proceeded to the two previous phases, it is the best time to take supplements that act directly on trigeminal neuralgia...
I propose a battery of the best natural supplements to fight this disease. Once the liver has been cleansed of toxins and heavy metals, these supplements become even more powerful.

These three phases form the fundamental basis of the most effective treatment available to eliminate trigeminal neuralgia.
I recommend that you follow the indications to the letter and do not take any other supplements outside the list during its realization.

I then completed the 3 PHASE SYSTEM with the

PHASE IV: EMOTIONAL TREATMENTS.
This phase is not essential, but it is useful if you wish to deepen the treatment and give it a new impulse from a different angle. PHASE IV consists of 3 different treatments that can be applied together or individually.

- **BIO-NEUROEMOTION**
- **BACH FLOWERS**
- **CALIFORNIA FLOWERS**

And to conclude, I have listed 13 other complementary treatments, which are not mandatory. They are simply an addition if you want to speed up the process :

- **SCHÜSSLER SALTS**
- **CHINESE HERBAL MEDICINE**
- **HOMEOPATHY**
- **CLASSICAL ACUPUNCTURE**
- **ZONAL ACUPUNCTURE**
- **TUNG ACUPUNCTURE**
- **YAMAMOTO CRANIOPUNCTURE**
- **AURICULOTHERAPY**
- **BIOMAGNETIC PAIR**
- **OSTEOPATHY**
- **KINESIOTAPING**
- **AROMATHERAPY**
- **EFT-Tapping**

With this set of treatments, you will be able to reach all levels of pathology: the physical level, the biochemical level, the energetic/biomagnetic level and the emotional/mental level.

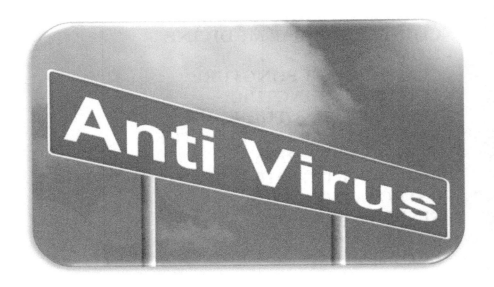

A virus is a piece of nucleic acid surrounded by bad news.

Peter Brian Medawar

The Liver, your Guardian Angel.

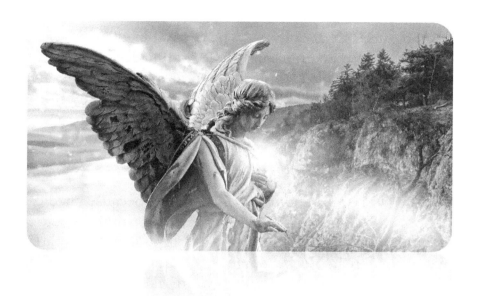

The liver is the third most intelligent organ after the brain and the thyroid. It is responsible for over 2,000 chemical functions and we are discovering more every day. It takes a lot of ingenuity to handle so much information. The stomach usually complains when it's not working properly, the intestines complain when they have pathology, the heart complains when it pumps irregularly, the lungs complain when they pick up harmful bacteria or a virus, the thyroid flares up when it's attacked by the Epstein-Barr virus... but the liver rarely makes its presence felt. It's a good thing it doesn't set off any alarm bells, because it's the front line. All the toxins that enter us through the air, skin, food and even radiation pass through it. It is responsible for purifying the blood so that these pathogens do not devastate your life. It is also the keeper of many viruses such as Herpes Zoster or Epstein-Barr virus which are responsible for countless diseases caused by neurotoxins, dermotoxins, viral corpses when combined with toxic heavy metals, radiation or DDT (herbicides, fungicides, pesticides). The liver stores these viruses deep inside and keeps them at bay, as long as it is healthy and strong. It is a tireless worker that performs a multitude of processes without which you would not be reading this book right now.

Doctors don't talk about the liver much because medical schools don't spend much time teaching future doctors about the anatomy of the liver and its constituent parts, unless you are a future surgeon or transplant specialist. Resources for general practitioners are like a few grains of sand on the beach. In fact, I don't know of a single drug that works for liver disease, as the drugs themselves are toxic and can only make things worse. Personally, I have suffered from liver inflammation on several occasions and the doctors have never been able to help me. As we have studied above, they are only prepared to administer drugs and there they are helpless.

The 6 main functions of the liver are:

- Process fats and protect the pancreas.
- Store glucose and glycogen.
- Store vitamins and minerals.
- Dismantle and immobilize harmful materials.
- Control and filter your blood.
- Protect you with its own personalized immune system.

The liver is the only organ in your body that is truly adaptogenic. It can switch from one task to another at breakneck speed and performs its various chemical functions without discussion, like a supercomputer. It is a born multitasker.

I won't go into the wonderful and exceptional nature of this organ, because that could fill thousands of pages, but I want you to be aware of its importance for your health.

Here is a series of pathologies that originate from a dysfunction of the liver:

- Appetite disorders
- Weight gain
- Gallstones
- Cancer
- Candida
- High cholesterol
- Dermatitis
- Dehydration
- Mood difficulties
- Autoimmune diseases
- Constipation
- Adrenal stress
- Lack of energy
- Strep throat
- Gout
- High blood pressure
- Gastrointestinal bloating
- Jaundice
- Sinus infections
- Gallbladder infections
- Yeast infections and bacterial vaginosis
- Inflammation
- Inflammation of the urinary tract
- Irritable bowel
- Liver worms
- Lupus
- Genetic mutations
- Mental fog
- Dark circles under the eyes
- Heart palpitations

- PANDAS
- Stomach problems
- Diabetes
- Aging problems
- Methylation problems
- Hormonal problems
- Rosacea
- Food sensitivities
- Chemical sensitivities
- Raynaud's syndrome
- Intestinal bacterial overgrowth
- Hot flashes
- Seasonal affective disorder
- Tumors and cysts
- Varicose veins
- Vitiligo

… to name a few, and of course Trigeminal Neuralgia.

We can divide this incredible organ into 5 specific parts:

- Center of the liver
- Lower part of the liver
- Upper part of the liver
- Left side of the liver
- Right side of the liver

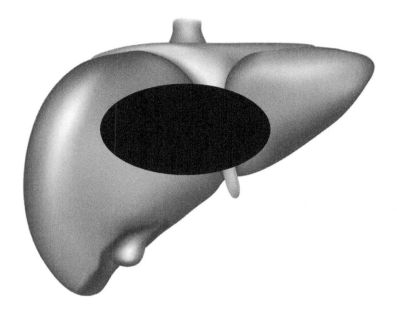

Center of the liver

A dysfunctional or sluggish liver in this area can result in symptoms such as: hot flashes, night sweats, onset of diabetes, bloating, water retention, body temperature changes, lack of energy, weight gain, mental fog, dark circles under the eyes, hypoglycemia, fatigue, rashes, anger, frustration, irritability, feelings of loneliness, depression, anxiety, distress, skin pigmentation problems or excessive thirst.

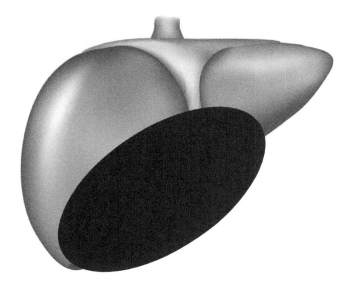

Lower part of the liver

A dysfunction of this part can lead to insomnia and sleep disorders, constipation, feelings of restlessness, feeling cold or hot contrary to the ambient temperature, jealousy or susceptibility.

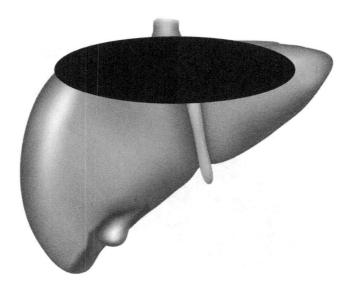

Upper part of the liver

Symptoms in this area may include: poor digestion, acid reflux, bloating, gastritis, pressure in the abdomen, irritability, frustration, stiff or sore shoulders, tongue sores, mouth ulcers, sores on the corners of the lips or in the mouth, fluctuations in body temperature, swelling or hardening of the upper stomach.

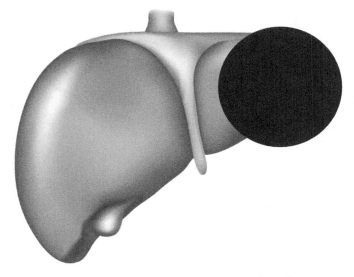

Left side of the liver

The sluggish left lobe can cause feelings of weakness in the left leg or arm, nausea, anxiety, lack of appetite, insatiable hunger, irregular stomach pain, mood disorders, irritability, emotional sensitivities and back pain.

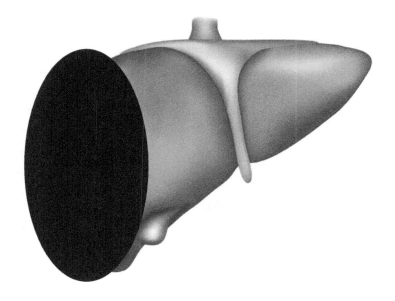

Right side of the liver

Right-sided dysfunction or laziness can result in brittle or discolored nails due to lack of zinc, stiffness of the ribs on the right side of the body, slight weakness on the right side of the body, spasms or cramps in the legs, slight discoloration of the tongue, irritation of the tip of the tongue, unexplained sensations of hot and cold, and difficulty warming up.

PHASE I: Liver cleansing

When we learn to drive, one of the first things we need to know are the danger signs to avoid problems. Knowing the prohibition signs, knowing what a red light means, recognizing that the cones on the road mean that there may be an obstacle, etc. In the same way, we will begin to recognize the things we need to avoid, the things that harm our implacable guardian angel.

These enemies of the liver can enter us by inhalation (we breathe diesel exhaust when we fill up the car for example), by contact (when handling poor quality plastics for example), by direct ingestion (food, water etc...), by direct exposure or even by radiation.

In many cases, it is virtually impossible to avoid them, but by being aware of these enemies, we can limit exposure to some extent and in others completely.

In order to be proactive in this regard, it is very interesting and important to be aware of these factors that aggravate our liver functions. These toxins that I will name below are the ones that cause the main functions of the liver to slow down or stagnate, causing dozens and dozens of diseases, including the high blood pressure that you are concerned about.

You should know that none of us are born with a 100% healthy liver, unless you were born in a remote jungle village, safe from the pollutants that plague us, and even then, some of them will get into your body, like radiation.

It is estimated that children are born with a liver at 70% of its capacity. Even if the pediatrician's office told you that you were one of the healthy ones, in reality, that is not exactly the case. And again, screening for a sluggish or toxic liver is not part of newborn screening. There are no studies on toxins in the child's liver received from the mother or father at conception. I am not talking about genes, but about toxic heavy metals, herbicides/pesticides/fungicides or DDT, viruses and radiation that are directly inherited and reside for years and years and generation after generation until one of the people in the family clan decides to do a liver cleanse.

In the baby, this results in colic, vomiting, unexplained diarrhea, just to name the most benign.

We continue to grow and perceive toxins everywhere. If our diet is not based on fruits and vegetables, it is almost impossible to get rid of so much waste and impurities and we will contract any kind of mild or fatal disease after years in an incomprehensible way. But let's not get carried away and focus on **the enemies of the liver.**

For this purpose, we must distinguish three different levels of organ depth:

- The perimeter surface (A)
- The subsurface (B)
- The deep inner core (C).

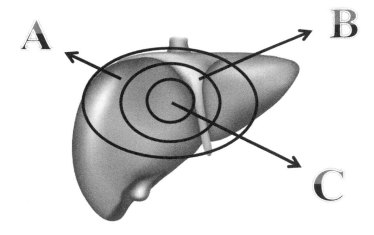

The enemies of the liver settle or are contained in it at one or more depths, often depending on how dangerous they are to you. The deeper they are, the more toxic and harmful they are and the harder it is to get rid of them. The more superficial they are, the easier it is to get them out of the liver.

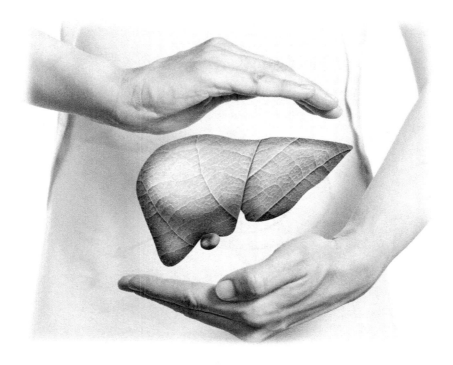

Every chemical that enters your bloodstream, whether through the lungs, stomach or skin, meets your liver at some point. The liver is your body's best defense when it comes to filtering out all these toxins, so you need to treat it properly.

Suzanne Somers

Enemies of the liver.

Petrochemical group:

The following products easily enter our body by inhalation or by direct contact with the skin if we touch them. They are extremely toxic to the central nervous system. They take a long time to leave the liver. The letters A, B or C indicate the depth at which they are generally installed.

- Plastics. (B)
- Gasoline. (B+C)
- Diesel fuel (B+C)
- Engine oil and grease (C)
- Exhaust gas (C)
- Kerosene (B+C)
- Cigarette lighter fluid (B+C)
- Stoves, grills and gas ovens (B+C)
- Solvents, solutions and chemicals (B+C)
- Dioxins (A+B+C)
- Lacquers (A+B+C)
- Paints (B+C)
- Paint thinner (B+C)
- Carpet and rug chemicals (A+B+C)

Neurochemical group:

The following products easily enter our body by inhalation or by direct skin contact if we touch them. Their hereditary factor is high. They strongly affect the central nervous system and getting rid of them is also a slow process.

- Chemical fertilizers (A+B+C)
- Insecticides, pesticides and herbicides (A+B+C)
- DDT (A+B+C)
- Fungicides (A+B+C)
- Fumes (A+B+C)
- Fluorine (A+B+C)
- Chlorine (A+B+C)

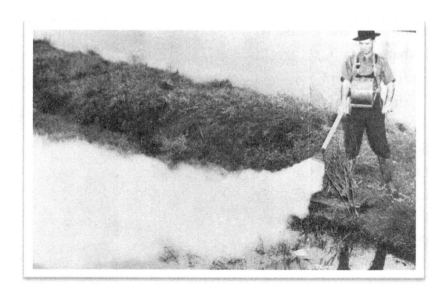

Problematic Food Chemicals Group:

The following products are easily found in countless baked goods, pastries and ready meals. It is easy to get rid of them by taking care of your liver (between 6 months and one year).

- Aspartame (C)
- Other artificial sweeteners (C)
- Monosodium glutamate (C)
- Formaldehyde (A+B+C)
- Preservatives (A)

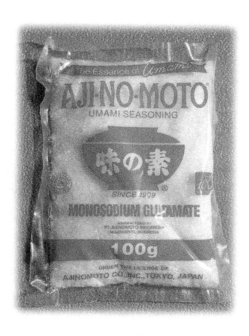

Risk food group:

These are the first things to come out of the liver if you take care of it. We will talk about this later.

- Eggs
- Dairy products
- Cheese
- Hormones in the diet
- Foods high in fat
- Alcohol
- Excessive use of vinegar
- Caffeine (A+B+C)
- Excessive use of salt
- Corn
- Canola oil
- Pork by-products
- Vinegar
- Soybeans
- Canned tuna

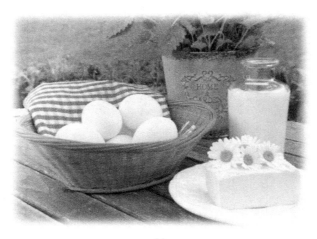

Group of pathogens:

Responsible for autoimmune diseases. Pathogens feed on any poisons they find in the liver. The solution to get rid of them is to eliminate their food sources. The time of elimination will depend on the aggressiveness of the pathogen, the duration of its presence in the body, the type of supplements you take and their regularity, as well as your diet.

- Viruses and viral residues (A+B+C)
- Non-productive bacteria (A+B+C)
- Toxins in food (B)
- Moulds (B)

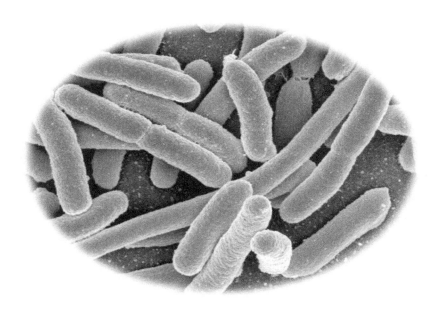

Household Chemicals Group:

These elements are very difficult to avoid because it also depends on the other people around us. They can start to disappear from the liver after a week and can be completely expelled within 3 to 6 months after the beginning of the cleaning.

- Air fresheners and scented candles (A+B)
- Deodorant sprays (A+B)
- Deodorant sprays and nebulizers (A+B)
- Colognes and aftershave lotions (A+B)
- Perfumes and lotions, creams, sprays, washes, shampoos, conditioners, gels and other conventionally scented hair products for the body (A+B)
- Hair fixative (A+B)
- Hair dyes (A+B+C)
- Talcum powder (A+B)
- Conventional make-up (A+B)
- Sunscreen spray (B)
- Nail chemicals (B+C)
- Conventional household cleaning products (B+C)
- Conventional detergents and fabric softeners and scented sanitary towels (A+B+C)
- Chemical products for dry cleaning (B+C)

Group of medicines:

Medications are necessary in the right measure. Some may save your life at one time, others (most) last too long and harm you. By taking care of your liver, some can take up to two years to leave your body, as they often contain oil. It depends on the drug and how long you take it.

- Antibiotics (B+C)
- Antidepressants (B+C)
- Anti-inflammatories (A+B+C)
- Sleeping pills (B)
- Biopharmaceuticals (A+B+C)
- Traditional immunosuppressants (A+B+C)
- Prescription amphetamines (A+B+C)
- Opioids (C)
- Statins (C)
- Hypertension drugs (B)
- Hormonal drugs (A+B)
- Thyroid drugs (A+B)
- Corticosteroids (A+B+C)
- Birth control pills (C)
- Alcohol (A+B+C)
- Recreational drugs (B+C)

Heavy metals group:

In Phase II, I intensively explain the problem of toxic heavy metals and where they are found. They can begin to leave the body within a week of starting the treatment. By applying Phase II chelation, you can completely expel them from the deep levels of the liver within one to two years.

- Mercury
- Lead
- Aluminium
- Copper
- Cadmium
- Baryum
- Nickel
- Arsenic

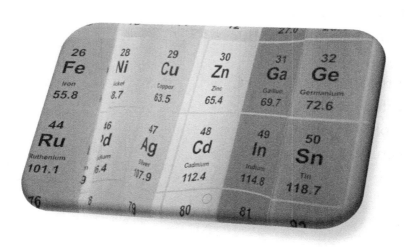

Radiation:

To these 8 groups of enemies of the liver, we must add the radiations that are found everywhere. Not only the radiation from the more than 2,000 nuclear explosions deliberately caused by the different military armies since the 1950s, but also the radiation in the air, in the water, in the soil and in our food. I should also mention the dozen or so nuclear power plant accidents in our history, as well as electromagnetic pollution from X-rays, scanners, cell phones, radioactive fallout and what you have inherited. Yes, radiation is inherited, just like heavy metals, viruses or DDT.

Radiation is deposited in all three levels of the liver. With the chelation program, you can get rid of all this contamination. The radiation particles start to come out after 3 to 4 weeks with the Phase II chelation system. It takes 1 to 3 years to completely clear. It all depends on how much exposure you have had.

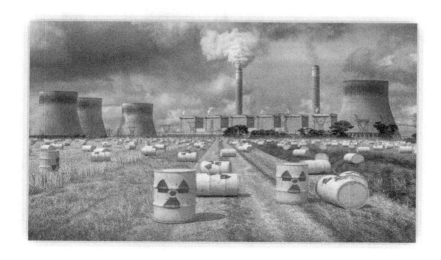

Excess of adrenaline:

- As I mentioned earlier, excess adrenaline also saturates our liver. We need to control prolonged **adrenal** stress over time. In addition, this hormone is a fuel for viruses and bacteria. Depending on the amount, it can stay at the B level or 3 levels deep. It can be eliminated in 1 to 3 weeks if you do a liver cleanse.

- **Adrenaline based activities also affect the liver.** All of these fashionable risk sports spike the adrenaline and saturate the liver on all 3 levels. It takes 1 to 3 weeks to recover from taking care of yourself.

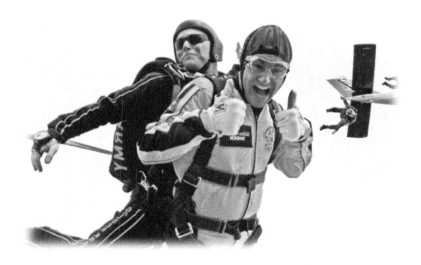

Once we are aware of all the negative factors in our disease, we are able to take action and at least limit our exposure to many of these harmful elements. Some are very simple, like putting on gloves when filling up the car and turning our face to the side so we don't absorb the fumes from the fuel. We can also wash our hands after carrying poor quality plastic bags. We can avoid lighting the barbecue fire with lighter fluid that will settle on the steak you are about to eat. Maybe you can avoid always cooking with gas.

Maybe you don't need to spray yourself with hairspray every day. You can buy organic foods with less fertilizer or other pesticides and insecticides. You can replace your aluminum or copper pots with ceramic or glass ones.

By avoiding diet drinks, you will reduce the consumption of sweeteners. Instead of eating 7 eggs a week, limit yourself to one or two. Dramatically reduce your consumption of dairy products and many aspects of your health will improve. Use lemon or orange juice instead of vinegar. Try reducing your coffee intake or eliminating it completely. Licorice root tea is a good substitute.

It is not difficult to reduce table salt consumption and there are many alternatives such as mountain rock salts. Replace rapeseed oil with sunflower or olive oil. Pork products are not good for you, replace them in part with other meats.

Don't buy air fresheners, and don't wear your favorite perfume or makeup all day, every day. Look for an environmentally friendly hair dye.

Family practitioners should be more concerned about liver health. Again, look for the original source, the primary cause, the origin of the pathology instead of treating the site of the symptom.

The problem with salt is that if we use refined, common table salt and abuse it, and if we consume a lot of fat, the fat in the bloodstream encapsulates the salt and produces denatured, dehydrated fat cells that eventually affect the liver. So reduce your salt intake a bit, but especially buy unrefined salt, preferably rock salt like Himalayan or high quality sea salt. The important thing is to reduce it.

Not all salts are bad, for example, the salts in celery are really medicinal. There are beneficial salts, like when we drink purified sea water, just as not all fats are so bad. You can't generalize like doctors or dieticians do.

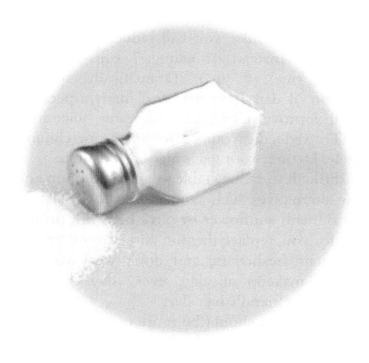

The problem with vinegar is that it is like alcohol for the liver, which becomes intoxicated and saturated, making it lazy and lethargic.

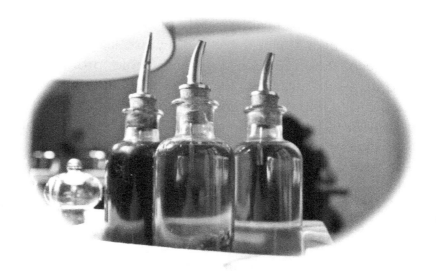

But you can tell me that you exercise, don't take fat, salt or vinegar and you have Trigeminal Neuralgia. In this case, the co-responsible party is toxins, which can be toxic heavy metals, viruses, viral waste, chlorine, fluoride or any other substance from the long list we saw above, turning your liver into a sluggish, clogged and stagnant organ. Anyone can have been exposed to these toxins, they are everywhere, or you may have even inherited them from your parents. Add to that the chronic dehydration we tend to experience, and you have all the ingredients.

And let's not forget stress, which forces our liver to eliminate all that excess cortisol or adrenaline. Never forget that **the virus is strengthened by the presence of these hormones**.

The problem with protein is that we have been fooled for almost 100 years. We have been led to believe that protein is just protein, and therefore beneficial, but this is far from the case. I am of course referring to animal proteins. Plant proteins are very healthy and bioassimilable. Animal proteins are high in fat, even if they are lean. And I say we've been deceived because this whole protein thing started in the 1930s. After the Great Depression, the large U.S. meat companies signed an agreement with the government to promote the marketing of all types of meat. A false propaganda campaign was launched, making us believe that protein is healthy and an alternative to fats and sugars. We were led to believe that sugars in fruit were bad and that the ideal diet was one high in protein (i.e. fat). People are often unaware that a diet high in animal protein is a diet high in radical fats. Nutritionists themselves are often misled by this misinformation when such diets are created. The result is further stagnation of the liver, an increase in pathogens and, in the long run, certain diseases from viruses that the liver is no longer able to contain or destroy. So if you want to increase your protein intake, look for it in vegetables, they are far more valuable, medicinal and bio-assimilable than animal proteins. Nutritionists are also wrong to say that, for example, 100 g of chicken breast contains 22 g of protein. Just as humans are all different, so are animals.

Some people have more fat, more muscle or more water in their body, the same goes for turkey, chicken or beef. 100g of turkey can contain 15g of protein or 30g depending on the poultry.

In any case, the meat to avoid above all is **pork, because it is the most contaminated** with all kinds of pathogens, hormones and drugs. It is also the fat that takes the longest to be transformed in the body, sometimes up to 10 hours longer than other meats. Processed meats are also a poor choice because they usually contain pork (radical fats), poor quality salts, dairy products, preservatives, smoke particles and God knows what else.

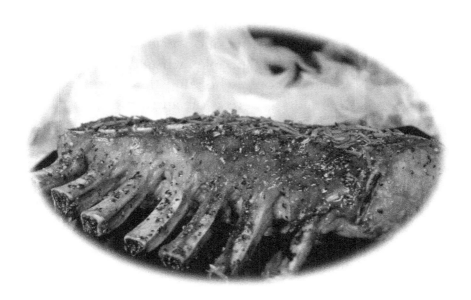

The problem with eggs is that they are one of those foods that we find hard to stop eating. There are many ways to prepare them (fried, boiled, scrambled, hard, beaten...) and they are usually incorporated in almost every dessert and pastry. We are often told that they are one of the best foods for our body, full of protein and energy. And that was true, a long time ago. It was true when our bodies weren't overrun with pathogens like they are today. Decades ago, our bodies did not have as many viruses, unproductive bacteria, toxic heavy metals, petrochemicals, plastics... (nor as many chronic diseases) as we have today. And it is precisely eggs that promote the viral explosion. It is the food that most favors the development of viruses. Don't believe them when they tell you that they are necessary and very healthy. The person who told you this probably doesn't have the right information or the most recent data.

You should know that all the publications you find about the benefits of eggs are information paid for by the food industry. Remember, the people who fund the food industry are the same people who fund the pharmaceutical industry and the media. There is an authentic story about eggs that you may not know yet and that will certainly surprise you...

Eggs were used as an abominable experiment in the not so distant past. This important survival food was taken and pathogens were created with it, which explains the high number of chronic diseases we have today. The truth has always been obscured. That surprised you, didn't it? I'll tell you how it happened...

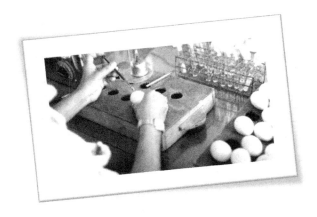

Decades ago, scientific laboratories grew pathogens by feeding them eggs. There they experimented with the viruses and bad bacteria that today produce most chronic and autoimmune diseases such as streptococcus, the herpes virus family, the Epstein-Barr virus family, cytomegalovirus, retrovirus, HIV, etc... In these eggs that served as food, they were manipulated and developed according to the whims of the "scientists" of these laboratories. These modified pathogens are now the cause of diseases such as cancer, multiple sclerosis, endometriosis, lupus, fibroids, polycystic ovarian syndrome, Hashimoto's thyroiditis or less serious diseases such as eczema, psoriasis, dizziness, vision problems, anxiety or depression, to name a few. It was known at the time that eggs were (and are) a good breeding ground for viruses and harmful bacteria.

All of this information from nearly 100 years ago was filed and patented by private laboratories to keep it out of the public domain and ignored by medical schools and doctors. Years later, leading virologists outside the health care system discovered the story through the various strains in the human body. This is how we learned that some of the worst viruses, such as Epstein-Barr or herpes zoster, were one of the worst artifacts created and spread by man, as a secret pandemic of multiple symptoms that medicine labeled as pathologies. With this story, I wanted to make you understand that we have been aware for almost a century that eggs are the perfect culture for the proliferation of viruses and harmful bacteria. Now that you have this valuable information, you will know what to do.

Once again, we see the deception of the pharmaceutical companies, the food industry, and medical manipulation. But unfortunately, we are not only fooled by the eggs...

The issue of dairy products is another important and serious one. Doctors, from pediatric offices to geriatric wards, have bombarded us with the importance of dairy consumption for the growth of babies, children, teenagers and into adulthood with the problem of osteoporosis and loss of muscle mass. Who doesn't like a glass of milk, yogurt with or without fruit flavoring, a good cheese or butter on bread?

If you are looking for a food for muscle mass, I am afraid it is not for you, because dairy products are not very bio-assimilable for the human body. Cow's milk is meant to feed a calf, not a human. This misconception that children should drink milk and yogurt is very old and the older the idea, the harder it is for a person to believe otherwise. Once again, we fall into the trap of doctors who recommend it and we believe it blindly, even though I prove it to you with the hundreds of studies that have been conducted and that confirm it.

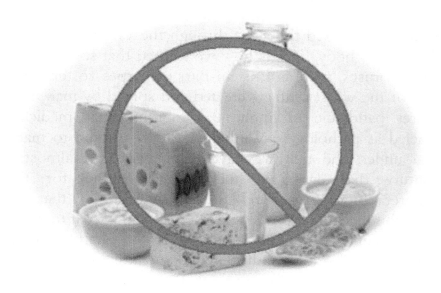

And if your goal is to prevent osteoporosis, you've been misinformed once again. Consumption of dairy products actually promotes the development of osteoporosis. Just look at the fact that in Asian countries, where milk consumption is almost non-existent, the rate of osteoporosis is practically zero compared to data from Western countries such as the United States where consumption is high. Milk acidifies the body and demineralizes it.

Several studies have shown that vegetarian women who do not drink milk have a bone loss rate of 18%, while non-vegetarians who consume dairy products daily have a bone loss rate of 35%.

The dairy industry is one of the largest in the food industry and just as they did in the 1930's with meat, they have also made people afraid not to drink milk. You know that a lie repeated over and over again becomes an unshakable truth. This industry leaves billions to the producers and especially to the pharmaceutical companies with the problems that come with it.

Cow's milk is high in fat and casein, a protein that is difficult for humans to digest. Milk can trigger allergic reactions such as asthma, ear infections, runny nose, colds, skin rashes, lethargy and irritability. In addition, some people lack the enzyme lactase, which breaks down the lactose in milk. If you really want to keep drinking it, switch to goat's milk or, better yet, grain-based beverages such as oats. This will give you much better calcium and protein absorption. Dairy products are big producers of mucus, and I'm sorry to tell you that this is no hoax. When you take milk away from children and replace it with cereal milk, the typical problems of phlegm, coughs, ear infections, allergic reactions, digestive problems, constipation and other associated conditions disappear. This milk has nothing to do with maternal milk, which is highly beneficial and nutritious. It has also been found that the arteries of children who drink cow's milk and its derivatives are in worse condition than those of children who do not drink it. Adults who try to eliminate it from their diet see improvement in many ways. Milk causes liver congestion, which is the cause of the mucus problem. Dairy products clog the digestive tract and allow pathogens to grow in the small intestine and colon. Unable to be properly processed by the body, they choke off essential oxygen. Dairy products also clog the lymphatic vessels and prevent the body from detoxifying naturally. Without proper cleansing, our pathogens will feel comfortable and proliferate. Eggs and dairy products aggravate chronic and autoimmune diseases. What's the point of seeking a cure for a disease if we are otherwise harming ourselves by eating harmful foods that contribute to it? If you get a cold, for example, the virus will have everything it needs if you eat milk, eggs or gluten; and these poisons will form mucus that will cause other problems such as coughing or nasal congestion. I should also point out that milk contains 59 different types of hormones that can cause a multitude of degenerative diseases. Its consumption is already associated with iron deficiency anemia, rheumatoid arthritis, osteoarthritis, asthma, autism, cataracts, ulcerative colitis, some forms of diabetes, Crohn's disease and coronary heart disease, multiple sclerosis, constipation, chronic fatigue, urinary incontinence, migraines, allergic reactions, sleep disorders, gastric ulcers, female infertility, lymphomas and various cancers.

Many people improve their neuralgia simply by giving up dairy products.

On the other hand, when you are in this first phase, trying to cleanse yourself, **avoid refreshments**. Most of them come in aluminum cans that release particles into the drink and we must specifically avoid toxic heavy metals as we will see in PHASE II. But that's not all, these drinks usually contain aspartame, corn syrup, flavoring and carbonated water.

All of these elements acidify the body and only slow down the work of the liver. Be aware that so-called "natural flavors" mean that they are made with monosodium glutamate, a very problematic compound. If they contain beet sugar, be aware that beets, like corn, are nowadays totally genetically modified.

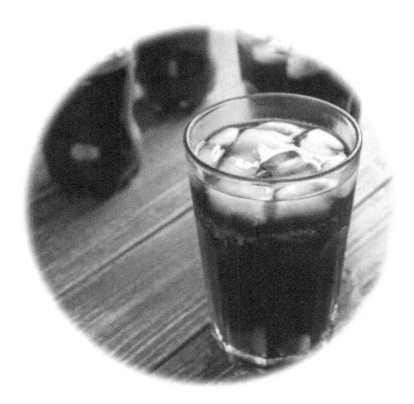

Another problem is tuna. It is often eaten in cans for its ease of use and good taste, but I regret to inform you that this is no longer a good choice. In addition to the toxic heavy metals you may have inherited from your parents at the time of conception (not in your genes), tuna will not only pick up aluminum from the can it is molded in, it also carries a lot of mercury, the most dangerous of the heavy metals. We will see in PHASE II but I can tell you in advance that mercury is responsible for countless pathologies such as autism, concentration difficulties, Parkinson's disease, memory loss, bipolar disorders and Alzheimer's disease.

If, in addition, it is associated with the Epstein-Barr virus, which almost all of us carry in our backpacks, we can associate it with diseases such as thyroid disorders, Lyme disease or all autoimmune diseases. Even worse, when the mercury in the tuna comes in contact with the aluminum can, a destructive interaction occurs that instantly creates a dangerous by-product. This combination is far worse than aluminum or mercury alone. Clearly, the problems don't come from eating a can of tuna, but if it's part of your regular diet, it can change your life, and you don't even know where the problem is coming from.

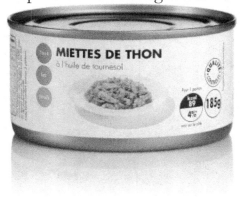

Be careful with arginine. L-arginine is an amino acid found naturally in red meat, poultry, fish and dairy products. It is needed for protein production and is commonly used for circulation.

L-arginine is converted in the body into a chemical called nitric oxide. Nitric oxide causes blood vessels to open wider to improve blood flow. L-arginine also stimulates the release of growth hormone, insulin and other substances in the body.

L-arginine is used to treat chest pain and various problems related to stroke, erectile dysfunction, high blood pressure during pregnancy and a serious condition in premature babies called necrotizing enterocolitis (NEC). It is also used for many other conditions.

It can be manufactured in laboratories and used in dietary supplements, and this is where the biggest problem lies. It is often marketed as a sports supplement to allow for increased vasodilation in the muscles, reduce fatigue and increase volume. It is a key component of many sports supplements.

The danger of arginine for you is that it is the opposite of lysine (which we will see later). In other words, while lysine kills the herpes zoster virus, arginine makes it extremely powerful.

As for corn, it is no longer consumable either, and I'm sorry if you like popcorn with a good movie in the theater. The corn that you find today is totally genetically modified, that is, transgenic. If you want to cleanse your liver of toxins, you need to avoid this food. Consider the fact that this corn is often fed to chickens whose eggs will end up on your plate. So here is another reason to put away the delicious eggs. In addition to genetic manipulation, they are full of fungicides and pesticides that will eventually saturate your body. I must admit that, like eggs, corn has also been used as an experimental base for breeding pathogens. So viruses and unproductive bacteria in your body love the presence of corn. This is a shame, because corn has been a great source of food for many people in the past.

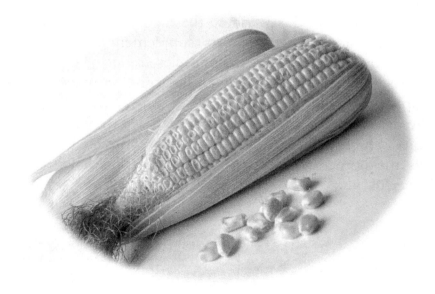

Unfortunately, the same is true for **soybeans**, which are now only available as GMOs and are loaded with pesticides, herbicides and germicides.

Here are some foods, herbs and supplements that are extremely beneficial to the liver. If you eliminate these pollutants as much as possible and incorporate these foods into your diet every day, your health will soon smile upon you. It is not a matter of consuming all of these supplements or foods on a daily basis, but rather incorporating each day one item from the list I am about to present to you.

These items will make it easier for your liver to do its hard work and fight off shingles and all the toxins that enter your body.

Hydration should never be forgotten. By default, humans are chronically dehydrated. In fact, we rarely drink enough for our bodies. Drinking plenty of hydrating fluids is crucial in the fight against neuralgia, not only because of the hydration it provides to the liver and other organs, but also because it is essential for getting rid of all the toxins that need to leave the body (neurotoxins, viral waste, viral corpses, etc.). It is necessary to help the lymphatic system by a good drainage through water and fruit or vegetable juices. Remember to drink a glass of water at least every two hours.

The Benefactors of the Liver

Therapeutic foods:

- Garlic
- Apricots
- Artichokes
- Atlantic seaweed (especially dulse and kelp)
- Celery (organic)
- Red bilberries
- Wild blueberries
- Berries
- Eggplant
- Sweet potatoes
- Broccoli
- Sprouts and micro greens
- Zucchini
- Winter pumpkins
- Onions and spring onions
- Cherries
- Cilantro
- Coconut
- Brussels sprouts
- Kohlrabi (kohlrabi)
- Turmeric (fresh)
- Dates
- Dandelion (leaves)
- Asparagus
- Spinach (organic)
- Pomegranates

- Peppers, or hot peppers such as cayenne, chili, habanero, jalapeño and poblano.
- Figs
- Maple syrup
- Kale
- Kiwi fruit
- Lemons and limes
- Red cabbage
- Mango
- Apples
- Peaches and nectarines
- Melons
- Honey (unpasteurized)
- Oranges and mandarins
- Papayas
- Potatoes
- Cucumbers
- Pears
- Parsley
- Pineapple
- Pitaya (dragon fruit)
- Bananas
- Radishes
- Rocket
- Mushrooms (organic)
- Tomatoes
- Grapes
- Cruciferous vegetables
- Green leafy vegetables (especially lettuce and lettuce stems)
- Carrots.
-
  .

Medicinal herbs and food supplements:

- 5-MTHF
- Wood sorrel
- ALA (alpha lipoic acid)
- Aloe vera
- Wild blueberry powder
- Ashwagandha
- Schisandra berry
- Amla berries
- Cardamom
- Milk Thistle
- Vitamin B complex
- CoQ10 (coenzyme Q10)
- Turmeric (in supplement form)
- Curcumin
- D-mannose
-EPA and DHA (elcosapentaenoic acid and docosahexaenoic acid) (without fish)
- Rosehip
- Spirulina
- Euphrasis
- Magnesium glycinate
- Glutathione
- Mullein
- Hibiscus
- Hydratis
- Raspberry leaf
- Olive leaf
- Nettle leaf
- Chaga mushroom
- Ginger
- L-lysine

- Melatonin
- Lemon balm
- Mint
- MSM (methylsulfonylmethane)
- NAC (N-acetylcysteine)
- American black walnut
- Chicory root
- Burdock root
- Dandelion root
- Licorice root (take for two weeks and stop for two weeks)
- Oregon grape root
- Selenium
- Red clover
- Cat's Claw
-Vitamin B12 (as adenosylcobalamin with methylcobalamin)
- Vitamin C
- Vitamin D3
- Nascent Iodine
- Zinc Sulfate
- Green barley juice powder

I recommend that you incorporate "therapy foods" into your diet every day. Try to eat one or more of these fruits or vegetables with each meal. If you are a picky eater, look for the ones you like best on the list and add them without restriction and enjoy them, knowing that each bite will rejuvenate and strengthen your liver. It's time to help your "guardian angel". You've been ignoring it since birth and it's time to pamper it so it can continue to support you until the last days of your life.
Choose at least 2 or 3 supplements from the list of "herbs and supplements" and incorporate them to give your best

friend a boost in healing. It will take at least a month for the decongestion to begin to resolve. In reality, the length of time will depend on many factors such as viral load, amount of toxic heavy metals, liver congestion, general inflammation, glucose, vitamin and mineral depletion.....

Remember one thing: even if your doctor has told you that you don't have liver problems, I remind you that a doctor does not have the training or the tools to perceive all the factors that cause chronic diseases. The proof is that you still have your pathology. Any good kinesiologist can give you a diagnosis with a high degree of reliability.

Instructions for liver cleansing:

1.   Avoid taking other supplements during the liver cleanse, such as protein powder, fish oil, collagen, chlorella, multivitamins, etc. If you continue to take supplements other than the ones I have suggested, you may not get the benefits you want.

2.   Celery juice is the best way to start.

3.   Then add vitamin B12 (with adenosylcobalamin and methylcobalamin), zinc sulfate, vitamin C (Ester-C or liposomal) or lemon balm.

4.   Then, if you can afford it, add spirulina, curcumin, cat's claw or L-lysine.

5.   If you don't get the result you want, modify or add to the list.

6.   Always choose supplements that do not contain alcohol. Alcoholic substances interfere with many of the properties of supplements. Remember that ethanol is an alcohol.

7.   Avoid supplements that contain too many ingredients in one. Too many substances in one product means that the quantity is too small.

8.   Look for quality supplements.

9.   You can mix these supplements without any problem.

The importance of celery juice:

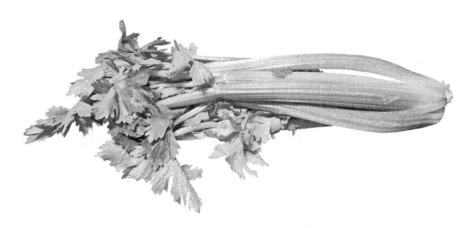

The first step is to drink celery juice every morning on an empty stomach. I recommend choosing organic celery, as this plant absorbs many of the toxins from the soil as it does from your body. Use a juicer to get all the juice. This plant has an incredible ability to make drastic changes on any disease. Therefore, you should drink it immediately on an empty stomach to get the full potential. This is the best way to purify the waste products that the liver has released into the various circulatory systems overnight.

It is important not to add anything else, no water, no lemon, no ice... Drink half a liter freshly squeezed and if you wish, half a liter in the evening.

If you don't have a juicer, you must cut off half a centimeter from the base of the celery stalk to separate the leaves and be able to rinse it. Then place it on a cutting board and cut it into pieces of about 3 centimeters, then put them in a blender until you get a smooth purée (without adding water). Strain the blended celery well. Wait at least half an hour before eating breakfast or anything else. The freshly squeezed juice retains its medicinal properties for about 24 hours.

Celery is one of the best anti-inflammatory foods available. It has the power to starve bad bacteria, yeast, mold, fungus and viruses and eliminate their toxins from the liver and intestinal tract. Eating celery is one of the best ways to alkalize the body.

.

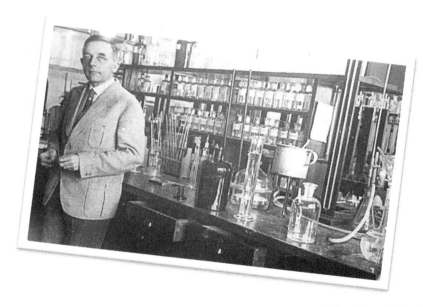

Dr. Otto Warburg

Dr. Otto Warburg, winner of the Nobel Prize in 1931 for the discovery of the cause of cancer, was very clear. He proved that there is no disease, including cancer, in an alkaline body. Of course, the pharmaceutical companies then made sure that people forgot about it, but we naturopaths always keep it in mind.

Well, as I said, celery is probably the best alkalizing agent you can find, and it's available in every supermarket and produce store at an affordable price. Many people improve their ailments simply by drinking celery juice every morning, without making any other changes.

If, for some reason, you can't drink celery juice, I recommend drinking lemon water. It is also a great alkalizer, a fantastic cleanser and a wonderful moisturizer. Prepare ½ lemon or 2 freshly cut limes with half a liter of water. Drink a pint just after waking up (to drain) and a pint before bed (to help the liver).

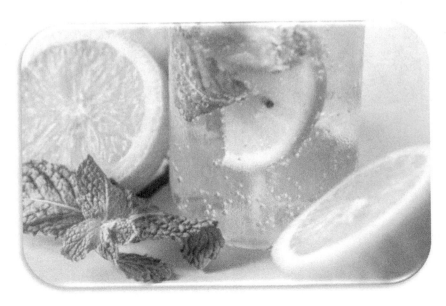

And if you really can't stand the flavors of celery and lemon, I recommend cucumber juice. It's also very alkalizing and hydrating, cleanses and purifies the body, and has a slight sweet taste that makes it easy to drink. Remove the skin from the cucumbers, unless they are from your own harvest, as they are covered in wax. Drink the juice of 2 cucumbers just after waking up. Cucumbers do not offer the same benefits as celery, so try to introduce celery little by little into your cucumber juice to get used to its taste.

I recommend that you avoid eggs, dairy products, gluten, canned soft drinks, excess salt, pork products, tuna, corn and all oils, soy, lamb, all fish, lamb, all fish and seafood (you can occasionally eat trout and sardines), vinegar, fermented foods (including kombucha, sauerkraut), caffeine, all grains (except millet and oats).

If you are able and want to give yourself a boost, completely avoid salt, radical fats, alcohol, natural and artificial flavors, nutritional yeast, citric acid, aspartame and other artificial sweeteners, MSG and preservatives.

Here is a 10 day liver cleanse diet if you want to go deeper into the cleanse. If you don't think you need it, try drinking celery, lemon or cucumber juice for a month, eliminate enemy foods and avoid other toxins. Add the beneficial foods each day and incorporate some of the supplements from the list.

10 Day Purification Regime.

Day 1	
Upon awakening	- ½ L lemon or lime water
Morning	- Normal breakfast - Mid-morning snack, if desired
Lunch	- Normal lunch
Afternoon	- 2 organic red apples - 1 to 4 dates.
Dinner	- Normal dinner
Before going to sleep	- ½ liter of lemon or lime water - Infusion of hibiscus or lemon balm.

Day 2	
Upon awakening	- ½ L lemon or lime water
Morning	- Normal breakfast - Mid-morning snack, if desired - 1 organic red apple
Lunch	- Normal lunch
Afternoon	- 2 organic red apples - 1 to 4 dates.
Dinner	- Normal dinner
Before going to sleep	- ½ liter of lemon or lime water - Infusion of hibiscus or lemon balm.

Day 3	
Upon awakening	- ½ L lemon or lime water
Morning	- Normal breakfast - Mid-morning snack at will - 2 organic red apples
Lunch	- Normal lunch
Afternoon	- 2 organic red apples - 1 to 4 dates
Dinner	- Normal dinner
Before going to sleep	- ½ liter of lemon or lime water - Infusion of hibiscus or lemon balm.

These first 3 days are intended to prepare the liver. It is not recommended to go on a deep cleanse without a minimum of preparation. It is comparable to the fact that if you are going to run a 100 meter race in a competition, you need to warm up first. It's never a good idea to rush in without warning. These three days are essential in order to move on to the next three days. You will have noticed that it is not very complicated and only varies by the amount of apples in the morning. Apples are an excellent food to cleanse the liver. If you do not like dates, you can replace them with dried or fresh blackberries, sultanas, raisins or figs.

It is important not to omit lemon water when you wake up to cleanse the impurities that have accumulated in the liver during the night. It is essential to incorporate more fruits and leafy vegetables than usual during these days. Avoid gluten, dairy products, eggs, lamb, pork and rapeseed oil.

Day 4	
Upon awakening	- ½ L lemon or lime water
Morning	- ½ L of celery juice - Super smoothie
Lunch	- Steamed asparagus with salad
Afternoon	- 2 organic apples - 1 to 4 dates. - Celery sticks.
Dinner	- Steamed asparagus with salad
Before going to sleep	- ½ liter of lemon or lime water - Infusion of hibiscus or lemon balm.

Day 5	
Upon awakening	- ½ L lemon or lime water
Morning	- ½ L of celery juice - Super smoothie
Lunch	- Steamed asparagus with salad
Afternoon	- 2 organic apples - 1 to 4 dates. - Celery sticks.
Dinner	- Steamed Brussels sprouts with salad
Before going to sleep	- ½ liter of lemon or lime water - Infusion of hibiscus or lemon balm.

Day 6	
Upon awakening	- ½ L lemon or lime water
Morning	- ½ L of celery juice - Super smoothie
Lunch	- Steamed asparagus and Brussels sprouts with salad.
Afternoon	- 2 organic apples - 1 to 4 dates. - Celery sticks..
Dinner	- Steamed asparagus and Brussels sprouts with salad
Before going to sleep	- ½ liter of lemon or lime water - Infusion of hibiscus or lemon balm.

As you will notice, there is no breakfast these days. The pint of celery juice will give you the nutrients you need and allow for more efficient elimination of toxins. If you feel hungry between the celery juice and lunch, have an apple or dates to fill you up. It's important that you never feel hungry - fruit or celery sticks are available to keep you from starving yourself. In fact, it's a good idea to have a snack every two hours to calm your adrenal glands. These three days can be the hardest because your pathogens will be hungry and will send you messages through your hormones to give in to temptation. You must resist, drink a glass of water every two hours and if you are hungry, eat an apple, dates, banana, pear...

What does the super smoothie consist of? (for 2 servings)

- 2 bananas or ½ papaya (preferably Maradol), diced.
- ½ cup fresh red pitaya (dragon fruit) or 1 frozen package or 2 tablespoons powdered.
- 2 cups fresh or frozen wild blueberries or 2 tablespoons powdered.
- ½ cup water (optional)

Another option would be:

- 1 mango
- ½ cup red pitaya, or 1 frozen package, or 2 tablespoons powder
- ½ cup sprouts (any spice)
- ½ lime
- ½ cup water (optional)

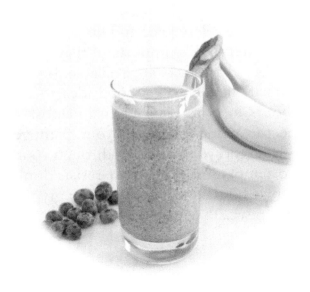

Here is the ideal salad for this diet, to eat at lunch and dinner.

Special salad for liver cleansing:

The quantities are for 2 to 3 people.

- 3 cups chopped tomatoes
- 1 cucumber, sliced, without skin
- 1 cup chopped celery
- 1 cup chopped cilantro (optional)
- ½ cup chopped parsley (optional)
- ½ cup chopped green onions (optional)
- 8 cups of a variety of green leafy vegetables (spinach, arugula, lettuce, etc...)
- Juice of one lemon, lime or orange.

You will see that there are many vegetables to choose from. It is important NOT to incorporate any type of oil as this will stagnate the liver and this diet will be useless.

Another option would be:

- 2 cups red cabbage, cut into thin strips
- 1 cup diced carrots
- 1 cup asparagus, cut into pieces
- 1 cup diced or sliced radishes
- ½ cup green cilantro, chopped
- 8 cups of a variety of green leafy vegetables (spinach, arugula, lettuce, etc.)

You can optionally dress your salad with orange juice, garlic, 1 tablespoon raw honey, ¼ cup water, 1/8 teaspoon sea salt, 1/8 teaspoon cayenne pepper.

It is important that these meals make you feel full enough, and don't worry about the calories, as they won't make you fat.

Day 7	
Upon awakening	- ½ L lemon or lime water
Morning	- ½ L of celery juice - Super smoothie
Lunch	- Cold spinach soup with cucumbers.
Afternoon	- 2 organic apples. - ½ L of celery juice. - Celery sticks and cucumber slices.
Dinner	- Steamed pumpkin, sweet potato or potato with asparagus and/or steamed Brussels sprouts, optional salad.
Before going to sleep	- ½ liter of lemon or lime water - Infusion of hibiscus or lemon balm.

A healthy look starts on the inside.

Robert Urich

Day 8	
Upon awakening	- ½ L lemon or lime water
Matinée	- ½ L of celery juice - Super smoothie
Morning	- Cold spinach soup with cucumbers.
Lunch	- 2 organic apples. - ½ L of celery juice. - Celery sticks and cucumber slices.
Afternoon	- Steamed asparagus and/or Brussels sprouts, and optional salad
Dinner	- ½ liter of lemon or lime water - Infusion of hibiscus or lemon balm.
Before going to sleep	- ½ liter of lemon or lime water - Infusion of hibiscus or lemon balm

Day 9	
Upon awakening	- ½ L lemon or lime water
Rest of the day	- 2 times ½ liter of celery juice (divided between morning and evening) - 2 times ½ liter of cucumber + apple juice (any time) - Melon smoothie, papaya smoothie or freshly squeezed orange juice (as often as you like) - ¼ liter of water minimum every 3 hours
Before going to sleep	- ½ liter of lemon or lime water - Infusion of hibiscus or lemon balm.

The spinach soup is cold, i.e. it is a smoothie so that it does not lose its properties when cooked.

During these 3 days, your liver will be releasing bundles of waste that you have been storing in the back of your liver for years, even decades. Drinking all of these fluids is crucial for hydration and especially for the overall cleansing of the body, providing it with a multitude of minerals, vitamins and medicinal compounds as well as a balance of carbohydrates. These last few days are focused on flushing out toxins, so don't be surprised if you have to go to the bathroom often. I recommend that you schedule this day to fall on a day of rest and devote it to total relaxation, your liver will thank you.

THE TENTH DAY, take it easy, start with the lemon water, then the celery juice and the super smoothie. You need to treat it carefully and incorporate the foods you want into your meals, except for fats and meats. Avoid the problematic foods we have seen and drink plenty of water. This is a transition day so as not to shock the liver and pancreas.

After these 10 days, you will notice unexpected changes in yourself. You will feel lighter, younger and more energetic. Many of your ailments will be gone or much reduced. In many cases, your neuralgia will already be balanced. And perhaps these rewarding effects will make you want to continue to eat healthily, and you will see other foods in a different light.

If you really can't do this 10-day cleanse for any reason, I recommend that you at least follow these guidelines for a month :

- ½ liter of lemon water at the time of getting up.
- Half an hour later, ½ liter of celery juice (cucumber + apple otherwise).
- 1 super smoothie in the morning.

Obviously, there are no contraindications, quite the contrary, and you can continue with these 3 instructions as long as you wish. Many of you will not need to go on to PHASE II and III after this treatment, especially the 10-day diet, because the cleansing is deep. This cleanse will also make you much less sick than before, as your liver will be rejuvenated and strengthened..

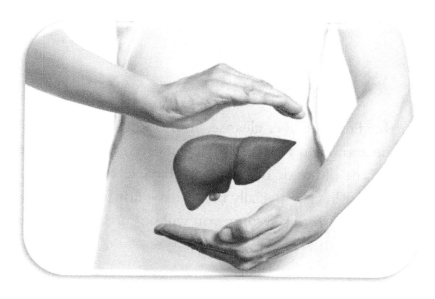

As I mentioned, this is the best method to date in terms of deep liver cleansing. **You should reject the following cleansing methods as they have been proven ineffective and have become old myths:**

- Eating bull's bile (your liver does not tolerate the bile of another animal).
- Eating liver (you are introducing toxins from the animal's liver into your body)
- Flushing the liver and gallbladder with oil and Epson salts (oil causes the liver to collapse).
- Drinking apple vinegar or apple cider vinegar (all vinegars saturate the liver)
- Coffee enemas (it is extremely acidic, dehydrating, very astringent and too stimulating)
- Eating beets (they are currently genetically modified))

After this fantastic liver cleanse, your body is ready to continue and begin PHASE II, chelation. It is possible that not all of the old toxic heavy metals have left the deep center of the liver, especially if you have not followed the 10 day diet. With this system, you will be sure that you have eliminated them...

PHASE II: Chelation

Group→	1	2	3	4	5	6	7	8	9	10	11	12	13	14	15	16	17	18
↓Period																		
1	1 H																	2 He
2	3 Li	4 Be											5 B	6 C	7 N	8 O	9 F	10 Ne
3	11 Na	12 Mg											13 Al	14 Si	15 P	16 S	17 Cl	18 Ar
4	19 K	20 Ca	21 Sc	22 Ti	23 V	24 Cr	25 Mn	26 Fe	27 Co	28 Ni	29 Cu	30 Zn	31 Ga	32 Ge	33 As	34 Se	35 Br	36 Kr
5	37 Rb	38 Sr	39 Y	40 Zr	41 Nb	42 Mo	43 Tc	44 Ru	45 Rh	46 Pd	47 Ag	48 Cd	49 In	50 Sn	51 Sb	52 Te	53 I	54 Xe
6	55 Cs	56 Ba	* 71 Lu	72 Hf	73 Ta	74 W	75 Re	76 Os	77 Ir	78 Pt	79 Au	80 Hg	81 Tl	82 Pb	83 Bi	84 Po	85 At	86 Rn
7	87 Fr	88 Ra	* 103 Lr	104 Rf	105 Db	106 Sg	107 Bh	108 Hs	109 Mt	110 Ds	111 Rg	112 Cn	113 Uut	114 Fl	115 Uup	116 Lv	117 Uus	118 Uuo

*	57 La	58 Ce	59 Pr	60 Nd	61 Pm	62 Sm	63 Eu	64 Gd	65 Tb	66 Dy	67 Ho	68 Er	69 Tm	70 Yb
**	89 Ac	90 Th	91 Pa	92 U	93 Np	94 Pu	95 Am	96 Cm	97 Bk	98 Cf	99 Es	100 Fm	101 Md	102 No

The human body is not able to metabolize heavy metals that persist in the body. These metal particles can have powerful toxic effects. Chelating agents are elements that will remove metal ions from tissues, preventing and reversing their toxicity and increasing their excretion. These heavy metals are found in all parts of the body but have a certain predilection for organs, particularly the brain and liver. In fact, the term "heavy metals" is not correct, it should be replaced by "toxic metals". The main ones are mercury, lead, cadmium and arsenic. Some less heavy metals are also toxic, such as beryllium and aluminum.

The main source of toxic metals is pollution.

Chelation therapy consists of administering chelating agents to eliminate heavy metals from the body. These chelating agents will, in this case, be very effective natural supplements to undertake this task.

Dear reader, you should know that this therapy is of paramount importance to get rid of neuralgia because we all have these metals in our body and they harm us in one way or another. The good thing is that it's simple and you don't necessarily need a specialist, although it's always advisable. All you need to do is take the right supplements and find a qualified dentist to remove the old amalgams if you have them. If you do, you should definitely look for a dentist who uses the safe amalgam removal system

The Amalgam Safe Removal Protocol (IAOMT), developed by the International Academy of Oral Medicine and Toxicology, consists of 8 important points:

- **Keep amalgams cool during extraction.**
- **Use a high volume suction device.**
- **Provide an alternate source of air.**
- **Immediate removal of mercury alloy.**
- **Wash and change gloves.**
- **Clean patient immediately.**
- **Consider dietary support (spirulina, selenium, MSM, coriander...).**
- **Maintain clean air in the office.**

The entire scientific community agrees that mercury, whether elemental (metallic), inorganic or organic, is a very dangerous toxic substance.

The WHO and other international organizations emphasize that there is NO safe level of mercury, that amalgam is the most important non-industrial source of mercury contamination.

People who remove metal amalgam fillings must take certain precautions before and after each extraction for safety. Unsafe removal can increase mercury levels in the body by up to 1,000 times, worsening health conditions. The mercury in today's dental amalgam is about 50% of the weight of each filling. I will explain these precautions later.

This therapy may take the longest time, depending on the degree of toxicity, but if we don't do it, we will never be able to get rid of our disease. Think that getting rid of these toxins will not only help you with your pathology, but also with many others that may have been preparing to appear. It is not easy to protect yourself from these metals, they are found everywhere (in food, soil, water bodies like lakes or reservoirs, vaccines, cigarettes, e-cigarettes, tap water, polluted air, they have even been found in baby food). A diet rich in natural chelating agents is therefore an excellent choice for everyone.

I will mention some pathologies, which can be caused by the presence of **mercury in the body**:

- Decreased work capacity.
- Progressive fatigue
- Mild irritation of the nerves
- Inflammation of the nasal mucosa
- Decreased memory
- Decreased self-esteem
- Irritability
- Headache
- Catarrhal symptoms
- Generalized weakness
- Insomnia
- Decreased intellectual faculties
- Depression
- Frequent diarrhea
- Spontaneous crying spells
- Sensation of cardiac compression
- Tremors
- Infertility
- Sudden Infant Death Syndrome
- Skin rashes
- Acne
- Food allergy
- Chronic bronchitis
- Lupus erythematosus
- Crohn's disease
- Ulcerative colitis

- Endometriosis
- Alzheimer's disease
- Hypertension
- Muscle atrophy
- Vision and hearing problems
- Tachycardia, heart attacks
- Anemia
- Apnea
- Gastritis
- Cancer

The list is even longer, I have given only a few examples for illustration.

One of the reasons why toxic heavy metals are so harmful is that they are neuro-antagonistic, i.e. they disrupt and disperse electrical nerve impulses and cause nerve damage.

In this process, neurotransmitters react like old light bulbs or transistors, burn out and melt, which can lead to anxiety and depression.

We can find in nature several very powerful products to eliminate toxic metals.

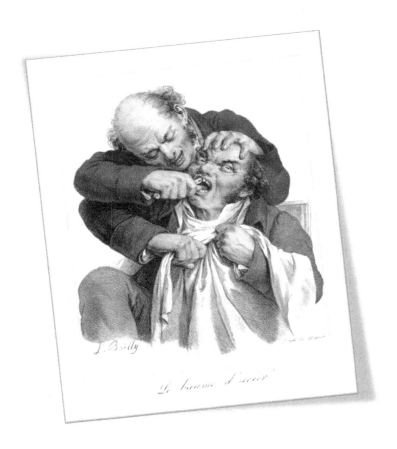

Dentist: a magician who puts metal in your mouth and pulls coins from your pocket.

Ambrose Bierce.

Today, it is common knowledge that **MERCURY** is toxic. But centuries ago, this was not known. Proof of this is that salts made from this heavy metal were used to treat syphilis from the 15th to the 19th century. It was also used as an antiseptic for wounds. Treatment can be administered orally, rectally, or by friction. The ointment made of mercury, lemon juice, pig fat, ash and oil was spread seven times [seven was a magic number] all over the trunk of the body.

Obviously, neither the Egyptians, who had a thorough knowledge of human anatomy, nor any other civilization knew at the time how harmful the use of this chemical element could be.

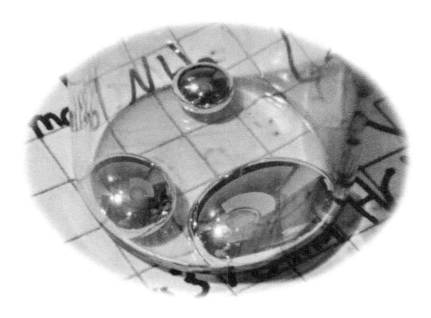

The Egyptians also came to use **LEAD**, another highly toxic element that can cause serious developmental disorders of the nervous system in children and heart problems in adults. In ancient Egypt, one of its derivatives, galena, was used to protect against the sun's reflection when it hit the sand. The black band with which they are represented in paintings is made of lead, which minimizes reflection.

Today, we can also be infected by lead: by having handled lead pencils as children; by being exposed to lead paint (either in the past when it was fresh or today when trying to remove it); by using water that has run through lead pipes in old buildings; and by having been in contact with pesticides, herbicides and fungicides.

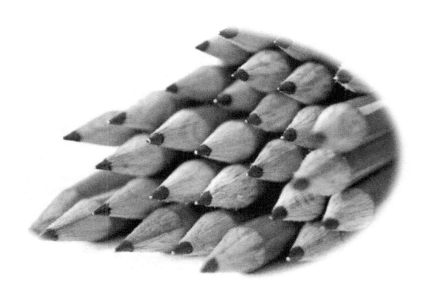

Another metal that is easily and increasingly entering our lives and our bodies is **ALUMINIUM**.

We are constantly in contact with it, from cans to aluminum foil, from ready-to-eat food containers to kitchen utensils, from make-up to deodorants, from tap water to sunscreens, from certain vaccines and medications to pesticides, herbicides and fungicides.

Pay attention to them in order to protect yourself as much as possible to save your liver.

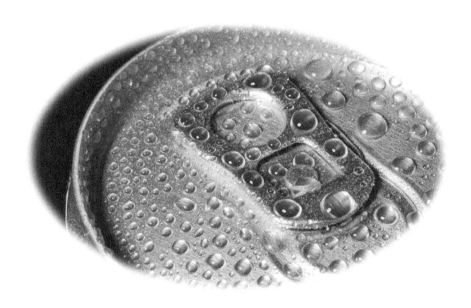

COPPER can also have a negative effect on the T.N.. The liver is very sensitive to it.

Copper is often used in plumbing, so copper particles can get into your drinking and bathing water, and it is often found in pesticides, herbicides and fungicides.

Copper pots and pans of all kinds are now in fashion in the kitchen; be careful and use ceramic pots and pans whenever possible; your liver and trigeminal nerve will thank you..

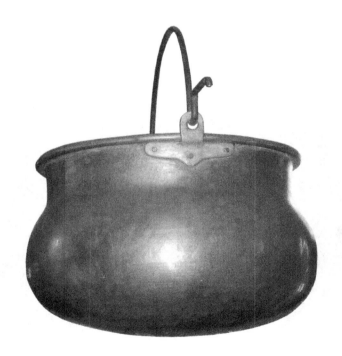

Another invisible enemy is **CADMIUM**.

It is in the air and falls from the sky, so it enters our bodies when we breathe. It is also present in pesticides, herbicides and fungicides.

It also causes:

- Diarrhea, stomach pain and violent vomiting.
- Broken bones.
- Reproductive failure, even infertility.
- Damage to the central nervous system and peripheral nerves.
- Damage to the immune system
- Psychological disorders.
- Possible damage to the DNA
- Development of cancer

.

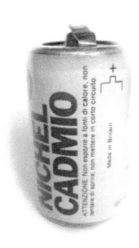

I will also mention **BARYUM**.

Another toxic heavy metal that affects our liver, preventing it from fighting the virus.

Barium is used in pyrotechnics. Metallic barium has few practical applications, although it is sometimes used to coat electrical conductors in electronic devices and in automobile ignition systems.

It is also found in pesticides, herbicides and fungicides.

It is in the air and falls from the sky, so it enters our bodies when we inhale it. We see how important it is to constantly clean our body and especially the liver.

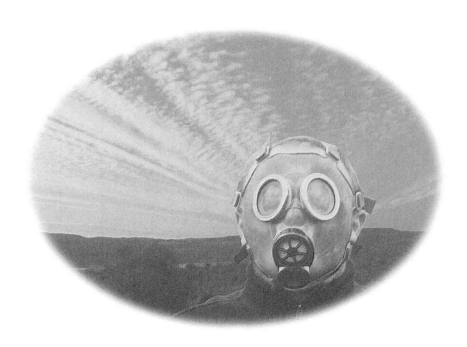

As for **NICKEL**, it is one of the ingredients of pesticides, herbicides and fungicides but it has other uses.

Pure nickel. Nickel, chemically pure or combined with very small quantities of other metals, is used in electronics and for the treatment of chemical products, especially in the chemical industry, and is used in nickel plating.

Nickel is applied to a variety of products through a process called galvanoplasty.

Stainless Steel. Nickel is alloyed with chromium and iron to form stainless steel used for kitchen sinks, stainless steel cutlery and cookware.

Nickel and copper alloys. They also have many marine related uses where durable, corrosion resistant products are needed.

Many countries use it in the manufacture of coins.

First of all, it is important to consider that this element can enter our body through breathing, direct contact with the skin or even through the ingestion of food contaminated by nickel.

It mainly affects the respiratory and renal systems. As far as the latter is concerned, the ingestion of water with a high nickel content causes an irregular concentration of proteins in the urine. This, of course, creates an imbalance that greatly compromises the kidneys.

As far as the respiratory system is concerned, the greatest risk lies in exposure to breathing in highly polluted places. Especially in areas close to mines or factories where automotive activities take place. It is common for a large portion of nickel particles to remain in the air and enter the body through breathing.

This seriously compromises the cells of the lungs, alveoli and bronchi. This tends to trigger conditions such as chronic bronchitis, pneumonia and even lung cancer. This of course jeopardizes the quality of life of the individual and can even lead to death.

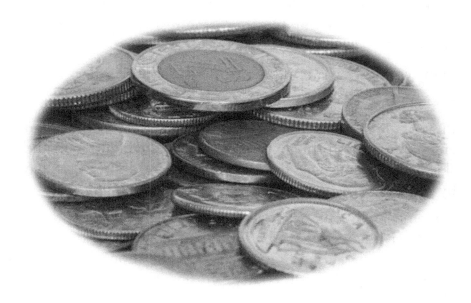

I will end these examples of toxic heavy metals with **ARSENIC**, another component of pesticides, herbicides and fungicides.

Metallic arsenic is primarily used to strengthen copper-lead alloys used in car batteries. It is also used in many pesticides, herbicides and insecticides, although this practice is becoming less common and is banned almost everywhere in the world. It has been used as a wood preservative because of its toxicity to insects, bacteria and molds, but it is also added to animal feed to prevent disease and promote growth. It is used in the medical treatment of cancer, such as acute promyelocytic leukemia, or in medical solutions such as Fowler's solution to treat psoriasis. Finally, this element is added in small quantities to alpha brass to make it resistant to zinc leaching. This type of brass is used to make plumbing fittings or other items that are in constant contact with water. In late 2009, the European Commission asked the European Food Safety Authority (EFSA) to conduct a new review of its levels and health effects. These are the ways arsenic is part of our lives.

It is also found in rice from India (mainly) and China (which is why rice is often called one of the 5 white poisons). To clean rice, it is necessary to soak it in water overnight.

Chelating foods and supplements

> ## Spirulina

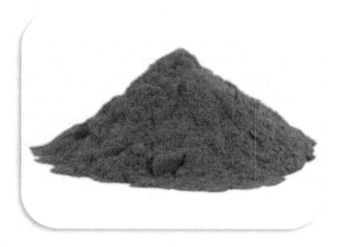

Spirulina provides us with a multitude of vitamins and minerals allowing the liver to store them for use when needed. This blue-green algae is able to stop viral and bacterial growth inside the liver and has the power to revitalize this organ by capturing hundreds of toxins and poisons such as toxic heavy metals and flushing them from the liver. It grows wild in warm water alkaline volcanic lakes. Today, we already have cultivated plantations and it is exported all over the world.

Spirulina has a high nutritional value, as 62-71% of the plant consists of essential amino acids. It is an important source of highly bioavailable protein.

I should also say that it is an excellent food against radiation exposure. It has very good results in terms of palliation of hair loss for people facing cancer treatments.

It is used for:

- Anemia
- Cancer
- Cholesterol
- Radioactive contamination
- Detoxification
- Immunity
- Hypertension
- Malnutrition and vitamin A deficiency

It is of interest to us in the case of trigeminal neuralgia because it provides the liver with a host of vitamins and minerals that are then delivered to the entire body.

Spirulina stops the herpes zoster virus and bacterial growth in the liver. The liver becomes more vital and regains the strength to draw out toxins in depth.

It plays a key role in strengthening the immune system of the liver and is involved in all its functions.

It also contributes to the storage of glucose and the reconversion of proteins.

DOSE:

2 teaspoons per day mixed with any liquid.

➢ Green barley juice powder

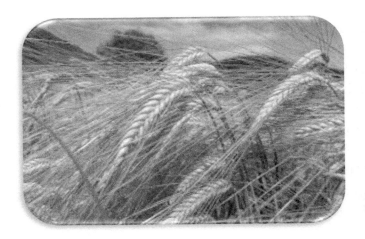

It is a true superfood. It contains phytonutrients that nourish the malnourished liver and allow it to detoxify from dozens of toxins and poisons inherited from the past and present. It removes toxins and replaces them with vital nutrients.

It is wonderful for facilitating the removal of mercury and other toxic heavy metals from the body.

When buying it, don't confuse it with green barley, look for **green barley juice powder**, it is more concentrated and contains many more nutrients.

This superfood has more properties:
Incredible alkalizer: it helps to maintain the acid-base balance of the body. Let's not forget that there is no disease in an alkaline body.
Strengthens the digestive system: helps fight heartburn.
Antioxidant: helps with skin problems (wrinkles, acne).
Helps the immune system.
Resolves halitosis and bad body odor.

DOSE :

2 teaspoons per day with water or fruit juice.

➢ MSM (organic sulfur)

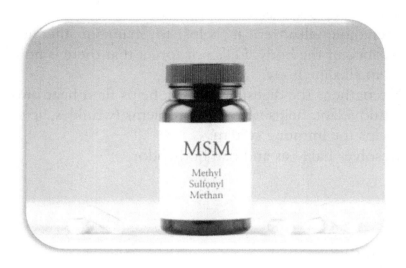

Methylsulfonylmethane (MSM) is a chemical substance found in green plants, animals and humans. It is a natural substance that is very effective against physical pain, especially osteoarthritis.

The sulfur provided by MSM is an excellent chelator of heavy metals.

Studies have shown that MSM can help purify the body by improving the permeability of cell membranes. It is a very good product for a detoxification cure. It also improves hair and nail health, helps protect the skin and has beneficial effects on allergies.

Recent studies show that taking this supplement may have anti-cancer potential, benefits for reducing snoring and positive effects on systemic lupus erythematosus.

MSM loosens fats from liver cells and helps expel them. This product strengthens the liver to fight bacteria and viruses. It also brings it out of stagnation and gently purges the gallbladder of small waste products.

It also strengthens the immune system in and around the liver.

It is recommended to take 5 or 6 g per day, on an empty stomach, meaning you can take a 2 g tablet on an empty stomach, another 2 g one hour before lunch and another 2 g one hour before dinner.

If you are being treated by a kinesiologist, he or she will be able to verify the exact amount your body needs with a simple test.

Nothing would increase the chances of survival on Earth like a switch to a vegetarian diet.

Albert Einstein.

> ## Coriander

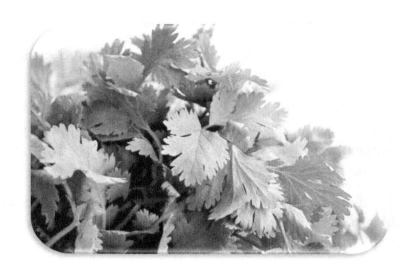

According to Dr. Yoshiaki Omura's research, coriander can effectively bind and remove mercury from our nervous system. It can also remove aluminum and lead. Daily consumption of coriander can remove significant amounts of heavy metals, within two to three weeks, through our urinary tract.

Coriander is quite anti-inflammatory and also has antiseptic properties. It contains 20% essential oils. This food, related to parsley, has a long tradition in the cuisine of Latin America, India and China. The origins of this plant, already mentioned in the Bible, are in the Eastern Mediterranean and the Middle East.

From a nutritional point of view, coriander provides us with vitamins C, K and A. It is also a source of minerals such as manganese, potassium, copper, iron and calcium, although not in very large quantities.

It is a powerful anti-cholesterol ally.

It will help to eliminate toxins from the liver. According to a study by the Autonomous University of Guadalajara (Mexico) and the University of California at Berkeley (California), this plant has antibiotic effects to break the membrane of the salmonella bacteria and weaken it until it is destroyed.

Coriander can reduce blood sugar and help kill certain parasites.

Other benefits of coriander:

- Alzheimer's Disease
- Senile dementia
- Depression
- Anxiety
- Obsessive-compulsive disorder
- Attention deficit hyperactivity disorder (ADHD)
- Autism
- Post-traumatic stress disorder
- Epstein-Barr virus infection/mononucleosis
- Herpes zoster
- HHV-6
- Cytomegalovirus infection
- Parkinson's disease
- Addison's disease
- Cushing's syndrome

- Postural orthostatic tachycardia syndrome
- Raynaud's syndrome
- Chronic fatigue syndrome
- Fibromyalgia
- Multiple sclerosis
- Migraines
- Vertigo
- Meniere's disease
- Thyroid diseases
- Ulcerative colitis
- Amyotrophic lateral sclerosis
- Eczema
- Psoriasis
- Urinary tract infections
- Insomnia
- All autoimmune diseases and disorders
- Fibroids
- Lesions

It must always be consumed fresh to obtain chelation, do not buy it as a supplement.

Food is a necessity, but it should only be consumed in the amount necessary to maintain the body.
If you exceed this limit, you will be faced with various problems.

Sathya Sai Baba

> **Garlic**

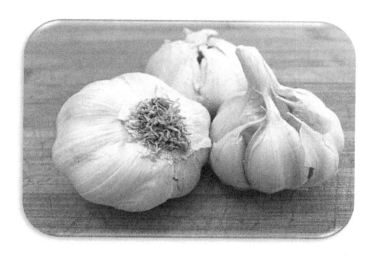

Garlic, which contains the chelating amino acids L-methionine and L-cysteine, mobilizes cadmium, lead, arsenic and mercury extracts in our body to eliminate them. Garlic is an ingredient that offers us a multitude of very interesting medicinal properties for our well-being. In fact, garlic contains more than 2,000 known active ingredients that help us maintain a stronger and healthier body.

Garlic acts as a natural antibiotic. In fact, it is rich in allicin, a property that acts as an antibacterial and will help us prevent the proliferation of bacteria in our body.

It is also an ideal ingredient to prevent the appearance of fungus in our body.

It has been proven that many fungal infections are sensitive to this food, because the extracts of the plant slow down the growth of molds and therefore prevent them from developing in us.

Some studies show that garlic can prevent the spread of certain viruses thanks to its antiviral properties.

Bad cholesterol (LDL) can clog artery walls over the years, so it is essential to regulate it and reduce its level in our blood. Garlic is a very powerful ingredient in this regard, as it works to regulate levels and reduce LDL. In fact, in the United States, many people consume garlic extracts to balance cholesterol.

Another of the properties and benefits of garlic is that it is an ideal natural remedy to reduce blood pressure and make blood circulation more fluid. This is because it helps to produce more nitric acid, a component that further dilutes the blood and thus helps to lower blood pressure.

Garlic is also ideal for keeping the body in optimal condition and preventing cell oxidation. This is due to the many antioxidants present in garlic, which help neutralize free radicals and keep the body younger and better protected. Allicin is one of the most powerful antioxidants present in garlic and will help you achieve the following benefits.

It is also recommended for the following disorders:

- Streptococcal pharyngitis
- Streptococcal vaginal infection
- Acne caused by streptococci
- Yeast infections
- Urinary tract infections (bladder and kidney)
- Staphylococcal infections
- Oedema
- Hordeolum
- Ear infections
- Sinus infections
- Chronic sinusitis
- Immune system deficiencies
- H.pylori infection
- Colds
- Influenza
- Bacterial pneumonia
- Breast cancer
- Laryngitis
- Esophageal cancer
- Prostate cancer
- Lymphoma
- Epstein-Barr virus infection
- Thyroid disease
- Adrenal fatigue
- Migraines
- Sleep apnea
- Lyme disease
- Psoriatic arthritis
- Eczema
- Psoriasis
- Herpes simplex

- Herpes simplex virus 1
- Herpes simplex virus 2
- HHV-6
- Infertility
- Pelvic inflammatory disease
- Ulcerative colitis
- Chronic bronchitis
- Intestinal bacterial overgrowth
- Thyroid nodules
- Thyroid cancer

Like cilantro, garlic is recommended for a multitude of conditions and can be classified as a medicinal food. As a chelating agent, I must also say that the latest research shows that it is NOT ONE OF THE BEST CHELATING AGENTS, but it is a wonderful superfood, so you can use it as a supplement for neuralgia.
Take one or two garlic teeth every night.

➢ Wild blueberries

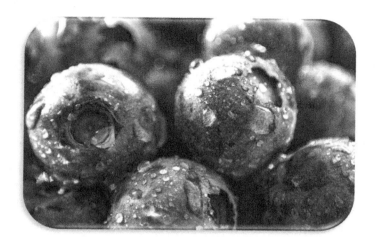

It is one of the most powerful foods in the world. There is no cancer that these berries cannot prevent and no disease known to mankind that they cannot protect you from.

Wild blueberries should not be confused with their cultivated relatives, which have far fewer benefits.

Today, nutrition experts recognize wild blueberries for their extremely high levels of antioxidants. But that's not all: they have the highest antioxidant content of any food on the planet.

When you eat these berries, their innate intelligence, built into their DNA, scans for possible illnesses, monitors your stress and toxicity levels, and designs the best way to heal you - the only food that can do this.

They are one of the most effective and wonderful foods for purifying heavy metals. They are the most powerful brain food, the most powerful prebiotic and a star of liver restoration..

If you eat them in a bowl with raw honey added, you get the most powerful prebiotic there is. If you take it shortly after sunrise, it will boost your energy and vitality throughout the day. Nibbling on a few handfuls of these wonderful berries between meals can raise your body's frequency and put you in a more positive and peaceful state. If you pick them from an organic garden or in the wild and eat them unwashed, you allow their high biotic content to restore the beneficial bacteria your gut so desperately needs and support your body's ability to produce all varieties of vitamin B12 coenzymes. Eating berries on a sunny day boosts adrenal gland strength and helps balance blood sugar. Eating berries on a cloudy day promotes liver cleansing and helps it wake up from its lethargy.

It powerfully accelerates the production of healthy liver cells and liver cleansing and regeneration. Incorporate it in your life if you suffer from any disorder (physical or emotional) and especially if it is cancerous, cerebral or nervous.

Consume half a cup a day.

> ➤ **Dates**

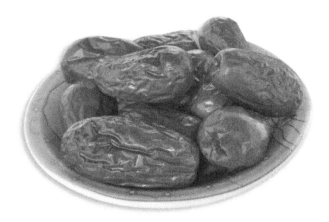

It is one of the most anti-parasitic foods in the world, adhering to parasites, yeasts, molds, fungi, candida, unproductive bacteria, viruses and heavy metals.

It is rich in over 60 bioactive minerals that support the adrenals.

It is one of the healthiest foods for the heart and contains a multitude of amino acids.

As if that weren't enough, it has abundant anti-cancer properties.

Take 4 to 6 a day.

The best variety is Medjoul.

If you have trouble falling asleep, take one two hours before bedtime..

It is recommended for the following disorders:

- Diabetes
- Hypoglycemia
- Intestinal bacterial overgrowth
- Cardiovascular diseases
- Fungal infections
- Gastroesophageal reflux disease
- Hypertension
- Lung cancer
- Obesity
- Thyroid disease
- Aneurysm
- Post-traumatic stress disorder
- Narcissistic personality disorder
- Obsessive-compulsive disorder
- Adrenal Fatigue
- Phobias
- Chronic sinusitis
- Rosacea
- Schizophrenia
- Social anxiety disorder
- Autism
- Attention deficit hyperactivity disorder (ADHD)
- Tuberculosis
- Vertigo
- Eating disorders
- Insomnia
- Periodontal disease
- Oedema

> ## Figs

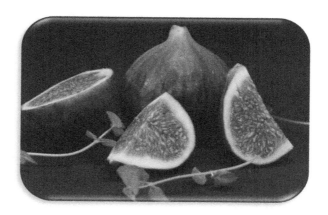

These fruits contain fantastic phytochemicals and plenty of potassium and sodium, which support neurotransmitters. Like dates, they are the best for cleaning the intestines. They not only rid us of heavy metals, but also of mold, unproductive bacteria and parasites.

Figs also cleanse us from radiation. They are very rich in B vitamins, trace elements, micronutrients, antioxidants, etc... Eat them with celery stalks to increase their medicinal power..

It is recommended for the following disorders:

- Alzheimer's disease
- Parkinson's disease
- Senile dementia
- Amyotrophic lateral sclerosis (ALS)
- Diverticulitis
- Wilson's disease

- Attention deficit hyperactivity disorder (ADHD)
- Epilepsy
- Salmonellosis
- Stroke
- Post-traumatic stress disorder
- Multiple myeloma
- Lymphoma
- Ovarian cancer
- Colon cancer
- Heart disease
- Bone cancer
- Chronic diarrhea
- Appendicitis
- Dyslexia
- Gallstones
- Urinary tract infections
- Postural orthostatic tachycardia syndrome
- Neuropathy
- E.coli infection
- Celiac disease
- Crohn's disease
- Eczema
- Psoriasis
- Hepatitis A
- Hepatitis B
- Hepatitis C
- Hepatitis D
- Megacolon
- Intestinal bacterial overgrowth
- Morton's Neuroma.

➢ Atlantic dulse seaweed

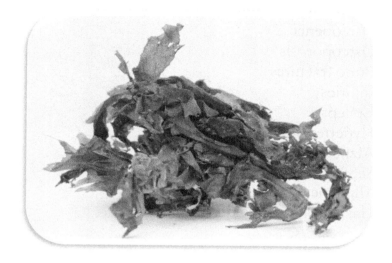

These algae have a huge potential to rid the body of toxic heavy metals. Notice if the consumption of these algae is important, that in the ocean, they are dedicated to absorbing toxic heavy metals, radiation, pesticides and other toxins and converting them into something harmless. Like dulse seaweed (the most powerful of all, as well as spirulina), I could mention bladderwrack, kelp, sea lettuce, laver or Irish moss, all have the property to transform these toxins and deactivate them.

In our bodies, what they do is that their substances take over these poisons and eliminate them from the body.

In addition to ridding the body of the worst toxins, these algae provide us with about 50 beneficial minerals.

Another great benefit is that it rebuilds damaged DNA.

It is very useful for the following disorders:

- Endocrine disorders
- Osteopenia
- Osteoporosis
- Bone fractures
- Injuries
- Epilepsy
- Hypertension
- Alzheimer's disease
- Senile dementia
- Migraines
- Hashimoto's thyroiditis
- Graves' disease
- Thyroid cancer
- Bipolar disorder
- Autism
- Attention deficit hyperactivity disorder (ADHD)
- Radiation exposure (from amalgams, x-rays or radiation therapy)
- Anemia
- Leukemia
- Bone cancer
- Brain tumor
- Bladder cancer
- Kidney cancer
- Liver cancer
- Lung cancer
- Stomach cancer
- Intestinal polyps
- Multiple chemical sensitivity
- Obsessive-compulsive disorder
- Depression

- Anxiety
- Parkinson's disease
- Reproductive cancers
- Asperger's syndrome
- Endometriosis
- Glaucoma
- Immune system deficiency
- Seasonal affective disorder
- Lupus

As you can see, the list of benefits is endless and we realize how many diseases are caused by the presence of toxic metals in our organs.

Tell me what you eat and I'll tell you who you are.

Anthelme Brillat-Savarín

➢ Apples

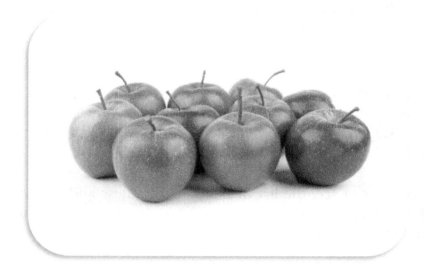

This fruit has tremendous anti-inflammatory power and can be recommended for almost any disease, just like wild blueberry.

It reduces the viral and bacterial load that creates these inflammations.

It is very nutritious for our brain as it nourishes our neurons and allows for better nerve connections. The flavonoids, rutin and quercetin that it possesses are responsible for the chelating action of this fruit and help eliminate radiation from the body. It also contains amino acids that rid your brain of the dreaded monosodium glutamate.

It is a true body cleanser. It also improves lymphatic circulation and regulates blood sugar.

It's the best thing for colon cleansing.

We are so used to seeing it that we ignore and underestimate its powerful benefits. But always look for organic and red. Non-organic products absorb too many pesticides, not to mention the wax they apply to increase their market value.

It is recommended for:

- Kidney diseases
- Liver diseases
- Alzheimer's disease
- Arthritis
- Seizure disorders
- Multiple sclerosis
- Thyroid disease
- Hypoglycemia
- Diabetes
- Transient ischemic attack
- Urinary tract infections
- Adrenal fatigue
- Migraine
- Herpes zoster
- Mould exposure
- Obsessive-compulsive disorder
- Osteomyelitis
- Attention deficit hyperactivity disorder (ADHD)
- Autism
- Post-traumatic stress disorder
- Acne
- Amyotrophic lateral sclerosis
- Lyme disease
- Intestinal bacterial overgrowth
- Anxiety

TRIGEMINAL NEURALGIA WITHOUT DRUGS

- Tinnitus
- Viral infections
- Dizziness

Try eating 3 apples a day and you will be surprised by the results in many aspects of your health.

Health is like money,
we never have a real idea of its value
until we lose it.

Josh Billings

➤ Melons and watermelons

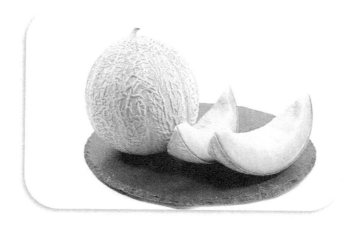

These two fruits are very important for people who are stuck in the healing process of an illness. They have an impressive digestive assimilation because they hardly need to be digested. Eating melon is like receiving intravenous nutrition, it goes almost directly to where it needs to go.

The juices carry and expel toxins such as molds, mycotoxins, viral neurotoxins, ammonia gas and bacterial toxins.

Its electrolytes protect us from strokes, aneurysms and embolisms. Melon liquefies the blood and reduces the risk of heart attacks and kidney and liver diseases.

If you want to alkalize your body, introduce melon in your diet, it is one of the most powerful.

It purifies the body from pesticides, herbicides and heavy metals present in the depths of the organs.

In addition, melon is ideal for ligaments, joints, bones, teeth, connective tissue and tendons because of its high silicium content.

It is recommended for:

- Infertility
- Crohn's disease
- Colitis
- Hypertension
- Peptic ulcer
- Barrett's esophagus
- Irritable bowel syndrome
- Aneurysm
- Embolism
- Stroke
- Myocardial infarction
- Kidney disease
- Breast cancer
- Pancreatic cancer
- Pancreatitis
- Tendonitis
- Epilepsy
- Sepsis
- Osteoporosis
- H. pylori infection
- Multiple sclerosis
- ALS
- Sjögren's syndrome

- Addison's disease
- Parkinson's disease
- Obsessive-compulsive disorder
- Attention deficit hyperactivity disorder (ADHD)
- Post-traumatic stress disorder
- Diabetes
- Hypoglycemia
- Acne
- Depression
- Anxiety
- Herpes infection
- Urinary tract infections
- Transient ischemic attack
- Heavy metal toxicity
- E. coli infection
- Yeast infections
- Mould exposure

Try to eat at least half a small melon a day, if that's too much, put it in a blender and juice it.
Don't eat it with heavy meals, have it in the morning with breakfast.

➤ Oranges and mandarins

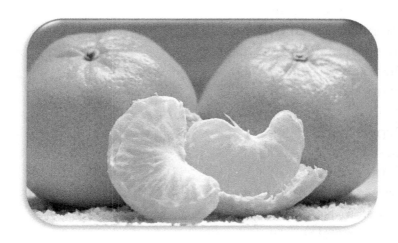

These fruits are full of the coenzyme glutathione, which is activated by their high content of flavonoids and limonoids. Let's not forget that glutathione is pure liver medicine.

These two fruits are the key to curing this century's epidemic of chronic disease.

These flavonoids and limonoids fight viruses, radiation and heavy metals in our bodies.

Oranges and mandarins contain a unique type of bioactive calcium. Contrary to the popular belief that the acid in these citrus fruits damages teeth, the opposite is true and it also dissolves kidney and gallstones.

Recommended for :

- Periodontal disease
- Kidney stones
- Strep throat
- Gallstones
- Osteoporosis
- Diabetes
- Hypoglycemia
- Mould exposure
- Adrenal fatigue
- Infertility
- Post-traumatic stress disorder
- Anxiety
- Depression
- Urinary tract infections
- Arteriosclerosis
- Stomach and intestinal cancer
- Acne
- Hypertension
- HHV-6
- Cytomegalovirus
- Herpes simplex
- Vhh-7
- Chronic fatigue syndrome
- Fibromyalgia
- Multiple sclerosis
- Lupus
- Graves' disease
- ALS
- Vertigo
- Lymphoma
- Epstein-Barr virus infection

- Hashimoto's thyroiditis
- Human papillomavirus infection
- Huntington's disease
- Herpes simplex 1
- Herpes simplex 2
- Bursitis
- Carpal tunnel syndrome
- Tendonitis
- Cold
- Nodules

I recommend taking 4 per day. If you take it with honey, you will increase by 50% the capacity of the pectin to kill and eliminate molds, yeasts, viruses and unproductive bacteria in the intestine.

Health is a state of complete harmony of body, mind and soul,
When one is free from physical ailments and mental distractions, the doors to the
soul open.

BKS Iyengar

HEAVY METAL CLEANER SHAKE

This shake is the perfect and powerful combination of 5 key ingredients for heavy metal cleansing and tastes great. These elements work in synergy with each other. It will not only rid you of toxic heavy metals, but also of radiation stored in your body and microplastics.

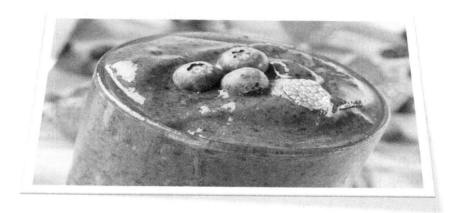

Ingredients for 1 person:

- 2 ripe bananas
- 2 cups of wild blueberries
- 1 cup cilantro
- 1 teaspoon barley grass juice powder
- 1 teaspoon of spirulina
- 1 tablespoon of Atlantic dulse seaweed
- 1 orange
- 1 cup of water

Place the bananas, blueberries, cilantro, barley grass juice powder, spirulina and dulse seaweed along with the orange juice in a high-speed blender and blend until smooth. Add up to 1 cup of water if you want a more liquid consistency. Serve and enjoy!

Tip: if the spirulina powder tastes too strong for your taste, start with a small amount and increase it.. Do not confuse barley grass juice powder with barley grass powder. Make sure the blueberries are wild (1000 times more potent than cultivated blueberries). Wild blueberries can be taken in powder form. Cilantro should be taken fresh.

This smoothie is what you should drink every morning, half an hour after drinking the water with the lemon juice, to cleanse yourself of the toxic heavy metals that are invading your body.

The time needed will depend on whether you have done the liver cleanse I explained in the previous chapter and on your toxic load.

You will find that this shake will improve many aspects of your health.

Try to consume it for at least 1 to 3 months for a radical change.

PHASE III: Antivirus

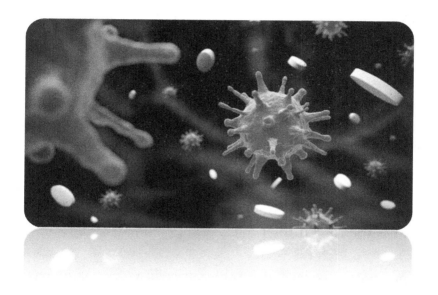

This section is of vital interest and one of the most important of all, because without it we could never enjoy full health. Unfortunately, our bodies harbor certain viruses, often encapsulated, latent, which are only waiting to manifest themselves if we offer them the desired conditions. The same viruses that make us sick can take up residence in the human body without causing a sneeze, cough or other symptoms. On average, healthy people harbor at least five types of viruses in their bodies, according to researchers at Washington University School of Medicine in St. Louis, USA. The researchers took samples from 102 healthy young people, aged 18 to 40, from five parts of their bodies: nose, skin, mouth, stool and vagina. At least one virus was detected in 92% of the subjects, and some had between 10 and 15 types of viruses. The reader can imagine what it would have been like if the entire body had been studied. Generally, our immune system is able to defend against them, but if they catch us off guard, such as poor diet, weak defenses, unmanaged emotions or dental amalgams, nothing can stop them. Scientists have found seven families of viruses, including strains of herpes viruses that are not sexually transmitted. For example, herpes viruses 6 or 7 were found in 98% of people. Anyone who has had varicella can develop herpes zoster later in life, even children. This is because the virus remains in their nervous system in an inactive (dormant) state for the rest of their lives.

Herpes zoster is caused by the varicella virus. After having varicella, the virus remains inactive in the nerve tissue near the spinal cord, liver and brain. Years later, the virus can reactivate as herpes zoster. Most cases of herpes zoster heal on their own, with or without treatment, and do not trigger other problems.

In very rare cases, herpes zoster can cause complications such as:

- Constant pain: Damage to the nerve fibers in the skin sends confusing messages to the brain, causing pain. This pain can last for a long time after the shingles have gone away. This is the most common complication of herpes zoster.
- Vision problems: If herpes zoster appears near the eye or inside the eye, it can cause vision loss.
- Skin infections: the shingles rash can be infected with bacteria, which can lead to impetigo or cellulitis.
- Nervous system problems: herpes zoster on the face can affect several different nerves that are connected to the brain. This can lead to nerve-related problems, such as facial paralysis, trigeminal neuralgia, and problems with hearing or balance. In very rare cases, it can lead to encephalitis (inflammation of the brain).

Antiviral medications cannot eliminate the virus from the body.
There are actually 31 varieties of herpes zoster and the one that affects the trigeminal area is the one commonly referred to as the "zona". These neurotoxins excreted by the herpes viruses cause various neurological symptoms or conditions. In the bloodstream, the neurotoxin is directed to adjacent areas where nerves are located. The herpes zoster virus that causes the dreaded trigeminal neuralgia leaves the liver and travels up into the jaw, into the areas where the trigeminal and even the phrenic and vagal nerves are located, enters the head area and excretes neurotoxins that are extremely allergenic to the nerves. So we need to pay special attention to the liver, because that is where it is

born and resides, where it hides, where it can lie dormant for decades.

If you have a lesion in the jaw, or a lesion in the area of those nerves, or if a dentist, for example, gives you a hard blow in the mouth, the virus is going to find that lesioned area and it's going to settle in that lesion and continue to work its way into the nerves,

releasing neurotoxins into the nerves.

Different levels of pain are due to different levels of toxins. Having rid the body of toxic metals through chelation, we have already taken a big step against herpes zoster. We have indeed deprived it of its favorite food. But we can deepen and eradicate its effects by removing certain foods from our diet, even if only for a short time, and increasing or adding new foods to stop it. It is possible that the trigger was a bee sting introducing a new toxin into your body, perhaps it was simply an excess of toxic metals; in all cases, we were able to demonstrate clinically that there is no trigeminal neuralgia without the herpes zoster virus.

I'm going to list a number of supplements that you should add to your diet to fight the virus (choose at least 5):

- **L-lysine**: 6 capsules of 500 mg twice a day.
- **Fresh celery juice**: increase to 1 liter/day.
- **Aloe vera**: 5 centimeters or more of fresh gel per day.
- **Yarrow**: 4 droppers twice a day).
- **Propolis** in drops or in infusion (very important)
(3 droppers 3 times a day)
- **Nettle leaf**: 4 droppers twice a day.
- **Licorice root**: 2 droppers twice a day (1 week long, 1 week off).
- **Propolis**: 3 droppers 3 times/day.
- **Vit.B12 (in the form of adenosylcobalamin and methylcobalamin)**: 3 drops 2 times/day.
- **Cat's claw**: 2 droppers twice a day.
- **Curcumin**: 3 capsules, 3 times/day.
- **Zinc sulfate**: 2 droppers twice a day.
- **Vitamin C (as Ester-C, Micro-C or liposomal)**: 8 capsules of 500 mg twice a day.
- **California poppy**: 3 droppers twice a day.
- **Lemon balm**: 4 droppers 3 times/day.
- **Spirulina**: 1 teaspoon or 3 grams/day.

In my experience, the best combination is:

- Liquid zinc sulfate
- Vitamin B12 (as adenosylcobalamin and methylcobalamin)
- L-lysine
- Lemon balm
- Cat's claw or licorice root

I put this arsenal of 18 supplements in case you can't find any or the price is too high. You can make any combination you like.

I recommend that you incorporate them into your life a little at a time to avoid the healing crisis that I will explain later.

Add one every 2 weeks until you are taking all 5 every day.

The drop tinctures should always be alcohol free.

When taking your supplements, pair them with a fruit, like a banana, or even a potato, sweet potato, pumpkin, dates, raw honey, pure maple syrup or coconut water. Natural sugar is what carries vitamins, minerals and other nutrients into the bloodstream and helps them find their way to their destination, and an organ will not accept them if it does not have this glucose.

As you can see, we have many weapons at our disposal. The length of the cleansing process depends on how long the virus has been in your body, whether it is in a healthy or toxic environment and the strength of your immune system.

It is essential to understand that it is as important to know what to eat as what not to eat:

Foods to avoid:

- **Eggs.**

- **All dairy products.**

- **Gluten.**

- **Soy.**

- **Pork**

- **Rapeseed oil**

- **Corn**

- **Arginine (often found in sports supplements)**

- **Natural flavor enhancers** (monosodium glutamate)

A diagnosis of herpes zoster is usually never made in the absence of a rash. In fact, the herpes zoster virus is responsible for the mysterious symptoms of millions of people, from unexplained skin rashes to neurological symptoms, migraines and more. There are eight strains of shingles that do not usually cause a rash, and neuralgia is one of them. Oral shingles, TMJ and Bell's palsy affect the gums and jaw. It is also responsible for Bell's palsy (viral inflammation of the facial nerves) and TMJ (the result of inflammation and pain of the trigeminal nerve). The neurotoxin travels to the larger nerves, so the internal pain and nerve damage is usually greater than with strains that cause rashes. It is very important to strengthen the immune system by eating well, exercising and getting enough sleep.

I have listed above a number of supplements that **help fight the virus,** but here are a number of foods that are also very helpful:

- **Wild blueberry**

- **Coconut**

- **Papaya**

- **Red skinned apple**

- **Pear**

- **Artichoke**

- **Banana**

- **Sweet potato**

- **Spinach**

- **Asparagus**

- **Lettuce (leafy and dark green or red varieties)**

- **Green beans**

- **Avocado**

These foods are helpful because they contain powerful phytochemicals that can attack different strains of the virus. This helps to recover from neurotoxins, boost the immune system, heal nerves, soothe inflamed skin and help detoxify the body.

Try, in Phase III, to incorporate one food from this list each day to support antiviral supplementation and save time on treatment.

SHOCK TREATMENT:

2 capsules of 500 mg vitamin C (Micro-C or alternatively liposomal or Ester-C) drained and mixed with a glass of water, 2 teaspoons of raw honey and the freshly squeezed juice of an orange every 3 hours as long as you are awake. If you do not have raw honey, you can use pure maple syrup.

Three Phases Summary.

PHASE I:

In my opinion, this is the most important phase. Just doing a liver cleanse can change your life and you may not need to do more. EVERYONE has a collapsed liver due to the poor intakes we use, so it will work for any pathology. Not doing a liver cleanse is like planting in an unprepared field. We need to pull the weeds, turn the soil and fertilize it if necessary. I highly recommend the 10 day diet. If you can't or don't want to do it, try for at least a month to drink the juice of half a lemon with half a liter of water twice a day. Then drink the organic celery juice. If you can't stand the taste, replace it with cucumber juice with apples. And if you want an extra boost, add the super smoothie. During this cleanse, avoid all the toxins we've seen, including fats (including meat and fish) if possible, vinegar and refined salt. Avoid eggs and dairy products. These products, as appetizing as they are, only make your life more difficult. Remember that they are often incorporated into many food products.

PHASE II:

During PHASE I, many toxic heavy metals will already be eliminated, but the oldest and most harmful ones will surely remain in the deep core of the liver. This phase is very manageable and ideal to implement right after the liver cleanse. Your liver is ready and strong to get rid of the last packets of waste. This phase can also change your life. Many aspects of your health that were bothering you will be resolved in no time. All you have to do is take the chelator shake in the morning. This shake is cleverly designed so that each element works together and works kinetically with the others.

Try to incorporate chelating foods each day during this time into your diet and continue with the PHASE I foods. If you continue to maintain a healthy liver, it will be easier for the liver to rid itself of toxins.

If you have metal dental amalgam fillings, I recommend that you replace them with composite amalgam fillings but follow the safe removal protocol. If you can't get your dentist to follow this protocol, take the chelation shake for at least a month after each extraction.

PHASE III:

If you've done the first two phases properly, you may not need any more. But if that's not the case, or if you want to be preventive, incorporate five supplements from the list into your daily routine. You can also alternate supplements as you use them. I recommend that you always have a basic one like vitamin B12 or zinc sulfate. Then add lemon balm and green barley juice, for example. The next month, replace the lemon balm with magnesium glycinate or spirulina, and so on.

Once you have been free of neuralgia for a while and your doctor has stopped treatment, continue to take at least one supplement a day to prevent a relapse. Zinc sulfate or B12 are excellent choices and will protect you from many diseases. With these two supplements, your liver's defenses will remain strong and it will be able to perform its countless tasks perfectly and continue to save your life, like the protective angel that it is.

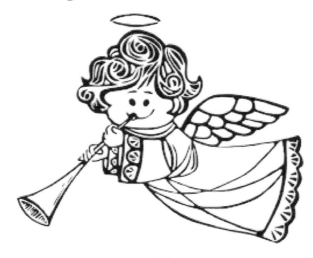

You have already learned how to take care of your liver and you know how important it is for trigeminal neuralgia. You now know the dangers that surround us all the time and directly affect it. You know the importance of toxic heavy metals and how to get rid of them and even avoid others. You have in your possession a battery of supplements and foods that improve your liver, repel metals and toxins, and neutralize herpes zoster. You have all the tools you need to create a new healthy body and free yourself permanently from a drug that will only make your problem worse, as we have seen.

Sometimes, some people may have uncomfortable or unpleasant reactions, both physically and emotionally, and we may think that the treatments or diet we are following is not working. These reactions are actually an expression that the body is responding to the given stimulus, and that the person is on the road to recovery. These reactions may last for a few hours or days, or even weeks, depending on the duration of the illness and/or its severity. Of course, as unique individuals, each of us will react uniquely and may have different reactions, with different intensities. It is even very likely that the same person will have different reactions at different stages, hence the importance of self-observation. In general, they tend to be more intense at the beginning of nutritional changes and detoxification, and as our bodies become more balanced, they tend to subside and/or disappear. My point is that **you should not be alarmed if you notice any changes that seem negative, it is simply part of the therapy.**

This reaction of the body is known as a **"healing crisis"** or **"Herxheimer syndrome"**.

Possible reactions may include the following:

- Headaches

- No more attacks for a few days

- Fever

- Cold or hot changes at night

- Excessive sweating

- Diarrhea, reflux

- Nausea

- Bloating and gas

- Abdominal pain

- Dry mouth

- Anxiety

- Fatigue, lassitude

- Sore throat

As the viral load decreases, viral waste products are released into the bloodstream, which tends to affect us in the same way as neurotoxins, causing the same pain. But you have to know that this means we have reduced the amount of important viruses, so you have to look at the positive side, even if it hurts for a while. This is why I insist on increasing fluid intake so that these viral wastes are not recirculated and reincorporated into the liver due to poor detoxification from dehydration.

I repeat that this is not always the case and that it is often the opposite that occurs, also bringing great vitality and well-being. These reactions are interesting because they are the symptoms that the toxins are mobilized and that the healing process is underway..

If a person wants to be healthy, they must first ask themselves if they are ready to eliminate the reasons for their illness.

Only then is it possible to help them.

Hippocrates

PHASE IV:

Emotional Treatments (optional)

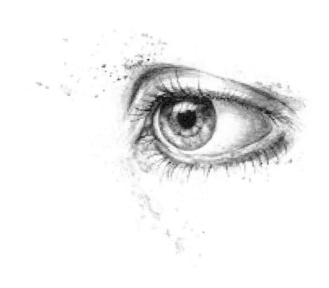

Anger, resentment and jealousy do not change the hearts of others, they only change yours.

Shannon L. Alder

Bioneuroemotion

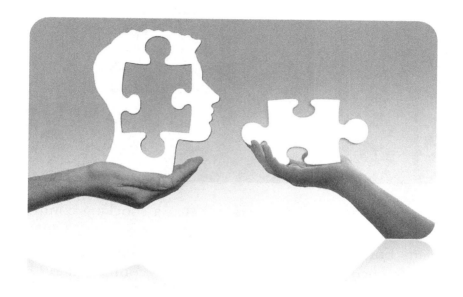

It all started with the German Ryke Geerd Hamer, a doctor of medicine and oncology, who in 1978, after the death of his son, developed cancer with his wife. They were struck by the fact that both cancers were related to the reproductive organs (his testicles and his wife's ovaries) and he wondered if this had anything to do with the death of his son, so he began to investigate, taking advantage of the patients in his practice.

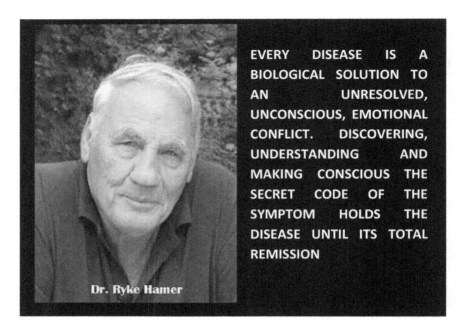

EVERY DISEASE IS A BIOLOGICAL SOLUTION TO AN UNRESOLVED, UNCONSCIOUS, EMOTIONAL CONFLICT. DISCOVERING, UNDERSTANDING AND MAKING CONSCIOUS THE SECRET CODE OF THE SYMPTOM HOLDS THE DISEASE UNTIL ITS TOTAL REMISSION

Dr. Ryke Hamer

The first thing he discovered was that a shocking conflict, i.e., trauma, experienced by the patient was related to an organ. For example, he discovered that his lung cancer patients had experienced a similar conflict and he wondered how this psychic conflict affected the brain. So he decided to study, by means of a scanner, if there were traces in the brain left by the emotional trauma. And he found circumferential spots in certain parts of the brain. He thought at first that they were the product of a machine error. He asked to change it and the same thing happened again, so he asked the patient to turn around, and the spot also turned around with him. No doubt the spot was not due to a malfunction of the machine but because it was actually in the brain organ. He then called this circumferential spot the "Hamer focus". He found that, for example, if 10 people had lung cancer, they all had the spot in the same place in the brain, and if 10 people had stomach cancer, they had spots in the same area between them, but in a different area than the previous group. This is how he made the first discovery of what he called "the iron law of cancer". At the same time, he also defined the type of conflict that the person must experience in order to develop a disease, since we all experience conflict all the time. He then notes that this emotional conflict must be a trauma, totally surprising and experienced in loneliness (not physical loneliness but emotional loneliness, that is, without the ability to share psychological pain). He concludes that the trauma lived in these conditions produces damage in the brain, then that the brain affects the organ that governs this damaged part, he thus finds a triad: psyche, brain, organ.

He continued his research and after studying more than 10,000 cases, in 1987, Dr. Hamer extended his discovery to all diseases known in medicine, under the name of the "Four biological laws". And in 1994, he added "The fifth biological law" which shows that disease is not a dysfunction of the human body, which is perfect, but an activation of special biologically significant programs that are attacks of the brain, whose only purpose is to release an emotional stress that threatens your survival or that of someone who is vital to your survival. Of course, conventional medicine turned its back on him, as it often does with geniuses, and proclaimed his studies dangerous. Now they will say that a discussion, delving into the unconscious, is dangerous! What will psychologists and psychiatrists say then? Science has always laughed at many things that turned out to be true afterwards and has assimilated them over time by appropriating the knowledge. I don't need to give examples, there is a multitude of historical facts.

What should be clear to us is that illnesses are not caused solely and exclusively by negative thoughts or poor emotional management. These negative emotions are triggers. That is, if the body is free of pathogens and toxins, emotions alone are not capable of producing that pathology. They will always be a kind of trigger if a virus, bacteria, mold, fungus or any other pathogen is circulating or hiding in the body. It will be the kindling for the fire. There is no fire without wood and oxygen. So that's what causes a disease to appear: it's almost always a pathogen with a trigger such as an emotion, toxic heavy metals, radiation or all the others we've already seen.

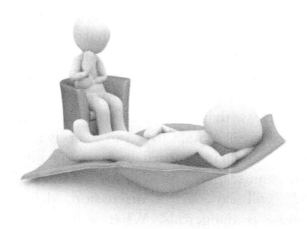

In my opinion, this could be a great step to start resolving a pathology. Indeed, negative emotions are burdens that weigh on our minds without us often being aware of it. The unresolved emotion is like a switch that we need to turn off. The difficulty is often knowing that the light bulb is on and burning us, and on the other hand we do not know where the switch is. Every disease is a lock in our unconscious and we have to find the key to unlock it. This is probably the hardest part to find on your own without the help of a specialist, but sometimes the simple memory is etched in your conscious mind and you know for sure that this is what it is all about. So I invite you to go back to your childhood, to the mountain of your memories, and think of something that has deeply affected you. This event can be physical, emotional or both. If you can't find that moment, your mind may have buried it in the memory trunk, but it never goes away, in fact, nothing goes away, everything goes into the subconscious. You can also ask for the help of a bio-decoder, a clinical hypnotist or a kinesiologist.

In any case, if you don't succeed, don't despair, the emotion will always be there but if you attack the disease with a good liver cleanse, chelation and supplementation, the result will be very effective. When I help my patients, I try to bring out the event that triggered their problem in order to deepen the healing and weaken it as much as possible.
Shocking negative emotions are burned into our brains, the so-called "Hamer focus", and the brain lets us know through illness, if the body meets all the necessary conditions, as we have seen.

What emotional conflicts are behind trigeminal neuralgia?

- A betrayal, a real slap in the face, even if it is expressed metaphorically.
- An aggressive separation, experienced either as a victim or as an aggressor.
- An attempt to escape a pain experienced in the past. When a current situation reminds him of that pain, he feels the same fears again, especially the guilt he felt at the time. An inner turmoil, full of bitterness, invades him.
- A punishment for a guilt. The anguish of communication.
- Self-deprecation, lack of self-esteem, not feeling capable of doing things, not feeling capable of taking on challenges..

The solution.

Once the cause is found, the remedy would be to face that pain from the past, to face the situation. Accept that you had boundaries at the time and that you have no reason to blame yourself or anyone else. It is important to forgive and forgive yourself, as neither side is to blame. Science now shows that forgiveness can have enormous health benefits, from relieving back pain to increasing athletic performance and even improving heart health. One study of a small group of people with chronic back pain found that those who meditated using forgiveness had less pain and anxiety than those who only received more frequent medical care. Another study showed that forgiving someone improved blood pressure and reduced heart overload. Studies on the impact of forgiveness conducted by Xue Zheng of the Rotterdam School of Management at Erasmus University have shown that forgiveness strengthens the body overall. In one study, participants even took a leap forward after writing about how they had forgiven someone who had hurt them and for whom they held a grudge. This is just one example of the importance of forgiveness. Guilt cannot exist because we all have recorded programs from our parents and ancestors or programs from our childhood that leave us guilt free. We have, unfortunately, a highly developed sense of guilt because of our educational system and we use it more than we should. We always tend to blame someone else for the things that happen to us when the only one responsible is us, you will have seen that I did not use the word guilty, but responsible. We have all, at one time or another in our lives, uttered sentences in which we blame ourselves or someone else. For example: "It was my/your/their fault".

And, while this is common, we may have gone too far in blaming ourselves or someone else for what is wrong.

The way we receive education, the way we perceive affection, the mother-child relationship, the father-child relationship will condition us from childhood and we will express it in the future. We already know, for example, that the relationship between a child and its mother will have repercussions on the relationships that this child will have with its partners once it is an adult. A bad relationship with the mother often translates into a bad relationship with women in the future. A daughter's poor relationship with her father will translate into a poor relationship with her boyfriend or husband in the future. No one is to blame, it is unconscious programming that is fixed in our brain. As children, we are constantly reminded of our bad behavior, and when we do something wrong, our parents are quick to tell us how disappointed they are in us. People are largely unaware of this inescapable effect. This guilt usually comes from family, friends, society or religion, which consciously or unconsciously teaches us to feel guilty for thinking or acting in a certain way. Ultimately, this practice is represented as social lynching. In fact, the feeling of guilt is so powerful that it is often used by governments to manipulate us. They always use a supposed act of another country or culture to disguise a war that actually has another objective, be it economic or power. They also use the bombardment of propagandistic news through the media to achieve the desired objective by blaming anyone who is in their interest. Guilt is indeed a very powerful weapon that must be handled with great care. This guilt can marginalize us, make us sick and even end our lives if we are not able to manage it.

Herpes zoster virus presents as small, very painful vesicles along the path of a nerve that has been damaged by neurotoxins. This infection is due to endogenous reactivation of the varicella zoster virus as a primary infection, which is very common in children. The Biological Sense is a protection in a situation of separation with the impression of being soiled, humiliated. We can therefore understand how, both in trigeminal neuralgia and in herpes zoster, there is an emotion of separation, of lack of protection. Often, finding the moment of the specific event in the past that triggered this emotion helps us a lot. Many people are cured for good. In most cases, the illness improves in a high percentage of cases. If it has not completely disappeared, I suggest the following exercise.

Solving exercise:

Redirecting emotions, turning negative emotions into positive ones, is the best way to improve the problem.

If you don't have the help of a specialist, I recommend closing your eyes and reliving the moment, as long as you have managed to recover the memory. Once you have found physical and mental relaxation in an alpha state (you can find alpha sounds on Youtube), if possible, relive the event as clearly as possible. In other words, try to see the colors, smell the smells and sounds. Feel it as if you were in the past, but exaggerate it. Amplify the pain you felt in that situation, but in the present. Stay a few minutes reliving the scene, somewhat exaggerated. Then, put yourself in the place of the person who hurt you, think about why he or she did it, what made him or her do it to you. Is it really his or her fault? Did he or she really want to hurt you? Think that something must have happened to him or to her as a child to make her act this way. A program in his or her subconscious must have caused her to make a mistake. Don't blame him or her for it, it was an unconscious lack of control. Now forgive him or her, imagine yourself hugging him/her and telling him/her that you forgive him/her, that you love him/her and that you understand him/her. Then forgive yourself for judging him/her and for hurting yourself because of that judgment. It wasn't your fault either, no one taught you to control your emotions

.

Bach Flower Remedies

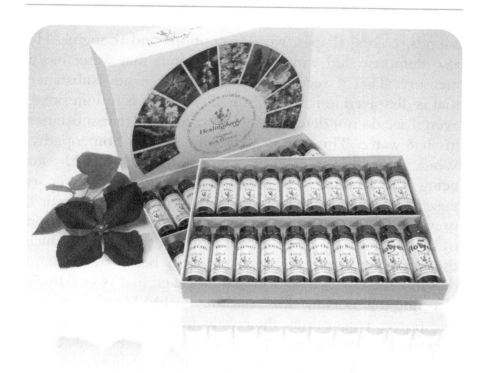

The British doctor Edward Bach, born in 1886, developed a system that, thanks to the essences of 38 flowers, manages to act positively on the negative emotions that affect our health. Based on the scientific fact that everything in the universe is vibration, including our body, the human being has a self-healing system that acts in the form of vibratory energy. The power of the flower essence lies in its energetic and vibrational qualities, which are able to affect our emotions.

The energetic information of the flower is transmitted to the water. The Japanese Masaru Emoto has demonstrated the power of water to transmit information and that the molecular structure of water records the vibrations of sounds, colors, shapes, words, emotions and thoughts. He also demonstrated with water ice crystals that water has a memory. That it records the vibrations of any substance that is dissolved in it, even if the dissolution is infinitesimal, even if we do not detect a single molecule of that substance in that water. This is the very principle of homeopathy. When these flower essences come into contact with our being, the vibratory frequency, as long as it is lower, is raised and aligned with the new vibratory frequency, preventing the effect of negative frequencies. The ingestion of these essences, carried by water, will correct and produce the energetic alignment of the person being treated and dissolve the energetic-emotional blockage that is negatively affecting that person, thus restoring health. Many therapists use flower essences as their only tool, as the results are spectacular. Based on the principle that behind every disease is a negative emotion and that every disease creates a new negative emotion, by changing the vibration of the emotion, we effectively solve the root health problem.

Masaru made an interesting experiment: he dissolved a drop of essential oil of cherry blossom in distilled water. He froze it and then thawed it slowly: crystals formed, visible only under a microscope, which he photographed and filmed. The water crystals curiously took the shape of the cherry blossom. He repeated the experiment with other flowers and the shape of the crystal always reproduced the geometry of the flower. He did another experiment with a Zen monk, giving him a vial containing water from a polluted lake that did not crystallize harmoniously, generating a deformed and ugly crystal. The monk meditates and projects his bliss on this bottle of water. When Masaru crystallized a drop under the microscope, he unfolded a very beautiful crystal. The monk's intention had modified its structure, giving it harmony. Thus, on a subatomic scale, water is able to capture and store the vibrations of emotions and thoughts.

The technology to detect these processes is not yet sufficiently refined. This is why scientists are silent. Although they already know that everything is vibration, it is information... In fact, quantum physics already speaks this language... But let's be patient, everything will eventually be proven.

Indications:

Flower essences can be found on the Internet, in some pharmacies or in herbalist shops. Once you have purchased the essences to take, mix **2 to 4 drops of the flower essence in a 30 ml dropper bottle of water, preferably spring water** (tap or bottled water is dead water, it has lost its vibration), and about 10 drops of vegetable glycerin. Glycerin is used as a preservative. It is possible to mix up to 7 different flowers in one bottle, although a maximum of 5 is recommended for maximum effect.

As this is a vibrational therapy, the success of the ingestions is determined by their frequency and not by their quantity. It is not herbal therapy, it is only a matter of provoking a certain impulse. This water, impregnated with the vibration of the flower, will in turn impregnate our body which is composed of 70% water to allow the resonance effect. **The frequency is 4 drops, 4 to 6 times a day, away from food and drink**. In case of severe crises, 4 drops every 5 to 10 minutes are recommended.

Advantages:

- No contraindications.
- They have no side effects.
- They are compatible with any other treatment.
- They have a holistic effect.
-They act on the energetic and vibrational levels.
- They are economical.

This therapy alone will not cure neuralgia in all cases, but it can play a relevant role, as it is the best emotional treatment and it is easy to use. This therapy will give a boost to others. In addition to the role of flower therapy in the prevention of emotional imbalance and its recovery, which has been progressively recognized since it was expressly mentioned by the World Health Organization in 1975, the possibilities of Bach Flower Therapy to act on different physical conditions are becoming more and more evident.

If you want to discover the secrets of the universe, think in terms of energy, frequency and vibration.

Nikola Tesla

Which flower to buy?

A simple way to determine which flower to take is to ask a kinesiologist using the Muscle Shortening Test (MST).
You can also consult a therapist who specializes in flower essences.
If you do not have the opportunity to visit one, you can easily rely on the following essences.

It is always a good idea to get a bottle called **Rescue Remedy**. It is not a single flower, but a compound of 5 flowers. I recommend it for emergency episodes, when the tension has gone up a notch.

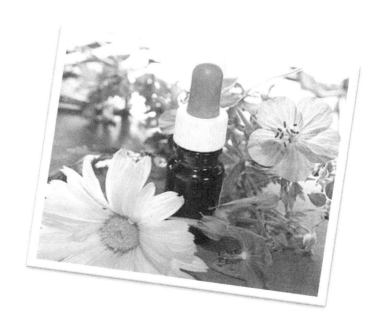

The five flowers of Rescue are composed of:

> **Rock Rose :** for the state of panic and terror caused by the crises.

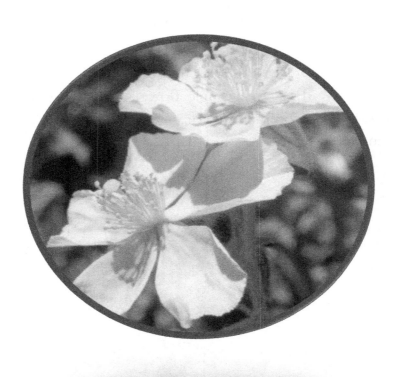

➢ **Clematis**: Helps to maintain contact with reality and in case of dizziness.

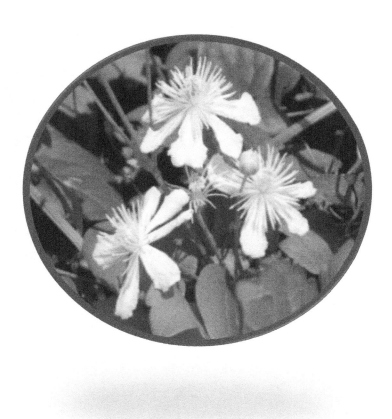

➢ **Impatiens**: for stress. Tension and pain.

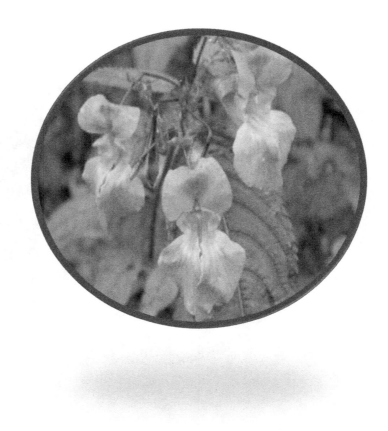

➢ **Cherry Plum**: to avoid loss of control or fear of loss of control.

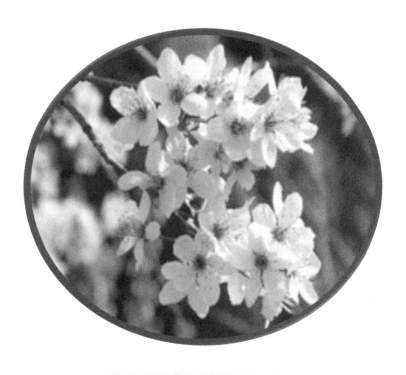

➢ **Star of Bethlehem**: synthesizes the action of the four previous essences. For trauma and restoration of the energy system.

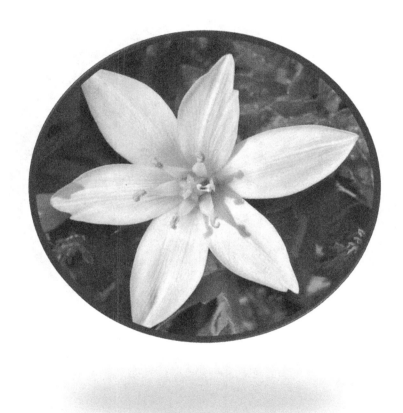

<u>In addition to the Rescue bottle for difficult moments, I
recommend a specific flower for trigeminal neuralgia:</u>

Beech:

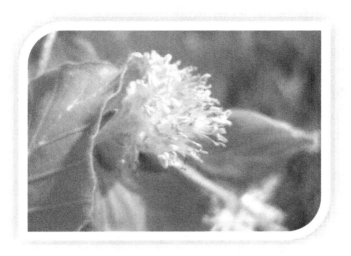

Beech is the archetype of intolerance, in the aspect of non-acceptance of the differences and imperfections of others and extreme sensitivity to their social or physical environment. It is intended for intolerant and critical people, who interfere in the lives of others without being able to put themselves in their place. They speak without knowing, they judge without knowing. They lack empathy. They are people who constantly see what others do wrong (in their opinion) and point it out to them at every moment, instead of seeing the positive aspects or virtues that everyone has. They don't take kindly to those who, in their eyes, behave in an unintelligent way, which is why they become annoying. They tend to be moody and cranky, although often what they criticize is not really important. They are often pedantic and inflexible, and often have a dominant personality. This essence helps one to be more tolerant and understanding of others, to find understanding, forbearance and tolerance, to understand that others can live according to their own system of ideals and to seek perfection accordingly. It shows us that each being, no matter how small, contributes to the whole, to the unity that we all are. From a physical point of view, it helps those who grind their teeth (bruxism) and tense their jaws and those with trigeminal neuralgia, when there is tension in the upper body or when the fists are clenched without realizing it, when noises are not tolerated and when there are ear or digestive problems. On an energetic level, it opens the heart chakra (fourth energy center).

<u>My recommendation is to mix 4 drops of Rescue, 4 drops of Beech, 30ml of spring water and take 4 drops, 4 times a day. In the acute phase, 4 drops every 5 to 10 minutes.</u>

The consumption should be done at least 6 months and up to one year after the last attack. It is recommended to keep the bottle away from electromagnetic sources such as cell phones, microwaves or Wi-Fi routers.

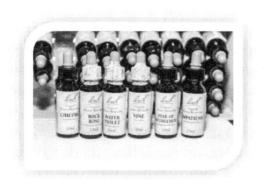

California Flowers Remedies

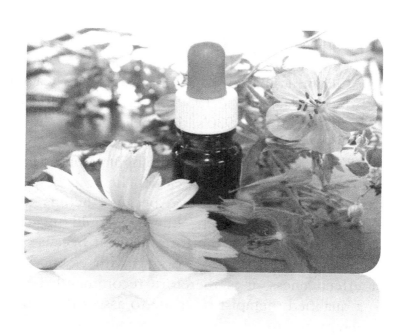

In the Californian Flower System, there are also essences that are successfully applied, reducing pain and improving quality of life. The principle is the same as that of the Bach Flowers seen previously.

California Flowers is a therapy that regulates different emotional and mental states by introducing positive archetypes into the person through certain flower essences.

Currently, the flower system is composed of 103 essences of different flowers, although it is considered an open system, that is to say, it is continually increasing, due to the new essences that are being experimented with and that are gradually included in the professional kit

Along with the Bach and Australian flower systems, it is one of the most recognized in the world and one of the most extensive and complete.

They were developed by the American couple: Patricia Kaminski and Richard Katz in the Sierra Nevada, in northern California, based on the discovery and teachings of Dr. Edward Bach (1886-1939), discoverer of the Bach Flower Remedies in the 1930's, thus belonging to the same therapeutic, energetic or vibratory system.

First of all, it is necessary to select the right essences for the preparation that I will present below. They can be chosen in a totally free and self-taught way because there is no risk of overdosing or side effects, but this could make one doubt the effectiveness of the formula itself because there is no previous experience of working with essences. For greater effectiveness, it is therefore recommended that a visit to a qualified therapist be made to assess the progress of the therapy and to select the essences to be included.

Second, 20-25% of the preservative, preferably vegetable glycerin, is placed in a 30 or 60 ml dropper bottle.

Third, the selected essences are mixed in the dropper bottle. 2 drops from the reserve bottle if you have a 30 ml dropper and 4 drops if you have a 60 ml dropper

Finally, complete the rest with mineral water (spring water if possible) and, after closing the bottle, shake vigorously to energize the formula. Never expose the flower essences to sources of electromagnetic waves (cell phones, microwaves, wifi, etc.).

Flower remedies are administered by taking 4 drops 4 to 6 times a day, on or under the tongue. It is important to keep in mind that the better the result, the more frequently the remedy is taken, rather than the amount administered. Therefore, if a more effective result is required at specific times, it is advisable to increase the number of doses per day.

Throughout the therapy, it is recommended that you become aware of changes in your responses to the topic you have chosen to work on. In some cases, you may experience immediate and truly dramatic changes, while others may have difficulty perceiving the changes. The most typical pattern is to discover a gradual effect over a period of time.

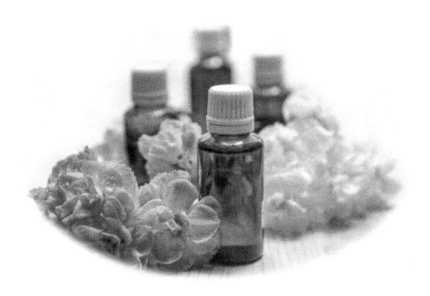

TORONGE

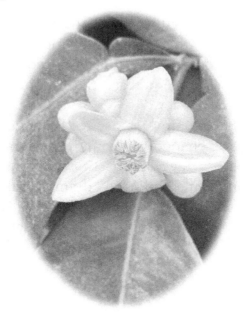

Toronja (grapefruit) flower essence works on imbalances in the head related to the jaw, temples, atlas (first cervical vertebra supporting the head), cranial plates and associated muscles. At the same time, more blood enters the head area to support the hair, face and complexion. It is an excellent complement to chiropractic, osteopathy, massage and craniosacral therapy to help realign the atlas, cranial plates and jaw line or to relieve headaches or TMJ (temporomandibular joint) disorders.

SNAPGRADON

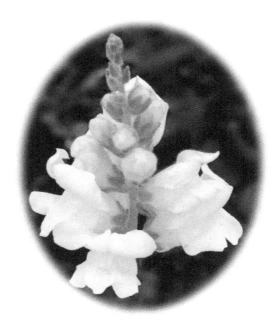

The essence of snapdragon acts on hostility, verbal aggression that you may have received at some point in your life or repressed emotions.

LAVENDER

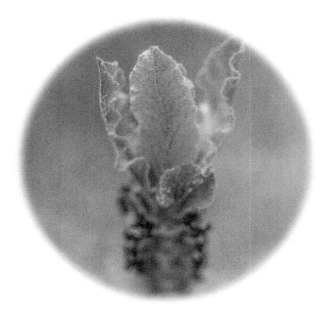

Used in cases of extreme sensitivity, exhaustion due to excessive sensory stimulation such as electric shocks.

ARNICA

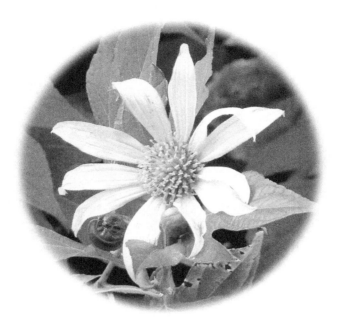

Arnica is mainly used in case of accidents and traumatic experiences as a trigger or secondary cause of T.N.

DOGWOOD

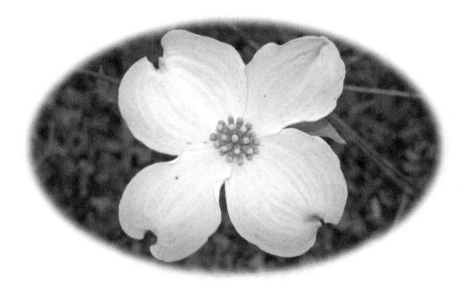

This essence is used in cases of unresolved emotional trauma, such as your N.T.

GOLDENEAR

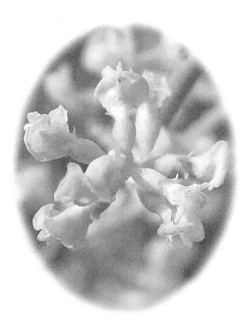

Goldenear is very similar to dogwood and acts on traumatic memories that affect current emotional life.

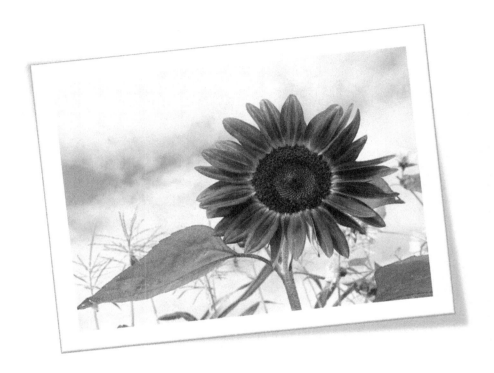

Everything in life is vibration.

Albert Einstein.

OPTIONAL COMPLEMENTARY TREATMENTS:

Schüssler Salts

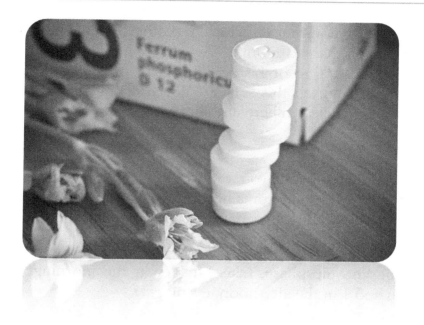

Schüssler salts are also called the salts of life. They consist of 12 minerals that are naturally found in our body through our diet. They are in fact functional, which means that each of them has a specific function at the right time and place. All of them, in their proper measure, provide energy and health.

These salts were discovered by the pioneer of biochemistry, Dr. Wilhelm Heinrich Schüssler, 130 years ago.

The scientist had discovered that by providing these substances, they could be much more effective than the pure minerals present in our food.

Schüssler's mineral salts can stimulate or restore bodily functions, and even correct functional disorders in the body. Although Schüssler spoke of salt molecules, it has been shown that mineral salts are created by the union of metals and non-metals, which take the form of ions and electrically charged atoms. I won't go into the details of their manufacture or history, there are many publications already written on this subject. You can find these salts in most pharmacies, in herbalist shops or on Internet.

How to take them?

In the acute phase, you can start with 1 tablet every 5 minutes. When symptoms begin to subside, the dose can be reduced to 1 tablet every hour, then every 2 hours, and finally 1 tablet three times a day.

In the chronic phase, take 1 tablet in the morning, 1 at noon and 1 in the afternoon/evening.

Children can take 1 tablet 1 to 3 times a day without problems.

The best way to take the tablets is to let them dissolve under the tongue.

The mineral salts are powdered salts containing lactose, they should not be taken by people who are allergic or severely intolerant to this ingredient.

In this section, I will only mention the salts that interest us for the relief of trigeminal neuralgia.

SALT N°4: KALIUM CHLORATUM

It is appropriate for:

Bronchitis, stuffy nose, skin rashes (eczema), inflammation of the stomach and intestinal mucosa, conjunctivitis, bursitis, arthritis and all inflammations caused by fever. It contributes to the medical treatment of first and second degree burns, inflammation of the tendon sheath, herpes zoster and dyspepsia.

We can see the importance of this salt in the fight against the herpes virus that affects the trigeminal area..

SALT N°5: KALIUM PHOSPHORICUM

It is indicated for :

This salt nourishes the nervous system and therefore acts on: mental, emotional and physical exhaustion, degrees of weakness (after stressful situations), insomnia caused by nerves, lack of energy, discouragement, cramps, localized alopecia and hyperactivity in children. It also helps to treat depression, muscle and heart weakness and paralysis.

In this case, the fact of being able to act directly on the nerves will be of a great help to calm the spasms, the state of anxiety and to be able to find the sleep.

SALT N°6: KALIUM SULFURICUM

It is indicated for:

All types of skin or liver disorders, for saturation of toxins in the liver and for all types of mucous membrane inflammations, for chronic rhinitis, and non-localized rheumatic pain. It also contributes to the clinical treatment of severe forms of the mentioned diseases, as well as psoriasis, depression and anxiety.

In this case, I advise it only to improve liver toxicity due to medication if this is the case and will not act directly on neuralgia.

SALT N°7: MAGNESIUM PHOSPHORICUM

It is indicated for :

It is the salt of the muscles. An additional help for sportsmen. It acts on muscle overload and cramps in the legs, stomach, blood vessels (such as migraine), painful menstruation and menstrual cramps, toothache, trigeminal neuralgia and children's stomach, asthma, muscle spasms, colic, insomnia, overexcitement, agitation, stage fright, test anxiety and nervous restlessness. It also reduces rheumatic pain. It also contributes to the clinical treatment of severe pain, cramps, kidney and gallbladder pain.

It forms a very good synergy with Salt #5 for neuralgia. It is another alternative to magnesium chloride or in its trace element form.

SALT N°12: CALCIUM SULFURICUM

It is recommended for:

Cellular cleansing treatments, suppuration of the skin and mucous membranes, growth disorders, chronic rheumatic problems, alterations in liver function, inflammation of lymph nodes due to swelling.

In this case, like salt n°6, we can use it in the hepatic cleansing due to medicines and cellular detoxification.

In summary, to counteract neuralgia, we can use salts n°4 (to attack the virus that produces it), n°5 (nerve) and n°7 (nerve).

If we have been taking medicines for a long time, we can use n°6 and n°12 for detoxification, especially of the liver.

But apart from these Schüssler salts, there is another excellent one, discovered later, which does not work with this company, called:

KALIUM JODATUM

It is used against all kinds of thyroid disorders, whether hyperfunction, hypofunction or goiter, i.e. it has a regulating effect on thyroid function.

It also has a pronounced effect on excessive nerve reactions, such as trigeminal neuralgia or sciatica. Also for headaches. In addition, it acts against inflammation, especially of the digestive system, and against inflammation of the eye. Very good for the mood like salt n°5.

It is also very useful for mucous membrane inflammations: respiratory tract. Acute and chronic rhinopharyngitis. Acne rosacea. Skin rashes. Chronic orchitis. Cervical adenitis (inflammation of lymph nodes). Tinnitus (ringing in the ears). Ocena. Atrophic rhinitis

Personally, it gave me **good results combined with Salt #5** during the acute phases. More than a salt, it is a homeopathic product, which could have a worsening of the symptoms at the beginning, then give way to an improvement.

I think the salts are a good tool, very economical, easy to take and combine very well with other treatments.

Chinese Herbal Medicine

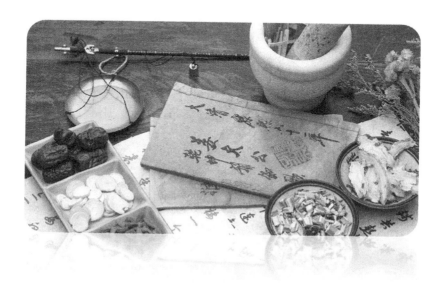

Chinese medicine is a very ancient therapeutic system, composed of acupuncture, herbal medicine and moxibustion, which, among other techniques, have developed together for more than 2,000 years. It is based on the philosophy of a civilization very different from ours, which perceives people as being "in harmony" or "in disharmony" with themselves and their environment.

Traditional Chinese Medicine (TCM) perceives illness in terms of disharmonious states and tries to restore balance in the sick person.

TCM uses different terms than the Western ones. Instead of talking about rheumatic or nervous diseases, it classifies pathologies as those caused by Wind, Heat, Humidity or Cold.

Instead of talking about rheumatism in the knee, we say, for example, Cold - Damp in the Stomach meridian.

Allopathic medicine focuses on a specific cause for a specific disease and when it isolates that cause or agent, it tries to control or destroy it. TCM also looks at the cause, but focuses on the patient's response to the disease entity, both physiological and psychological. In other words, it is much more comprehensive and considers the body as a whole (as it should be).

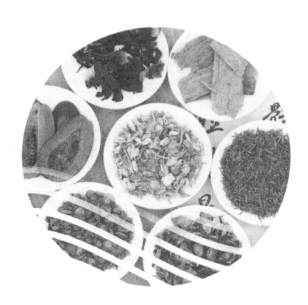

The treatment will be directed at the wind, moisture and heat that may have entered the meridians and produced the disease.

Chi (vital energy) is everywhere in the body, but it circulates through a few main channels, nourishing and warming the organs and other parts of the body and harmonizing their activity. These channels form what is called the meridian system (Jing-Luo). Most acupuncture points are found along these meridians and most herbs prescribed by a Chinese therapist penetrate one or more of them. There are twelve main meridians, which correspond to the twelve main organs and are named after them: Liver, Heart, Stomach, Kidney, Spleen, etc. These meridians are bilateral, that is to say that they appear in identical pairs, one on each side of the body. Some meridians are more yin, they have functions more related to the accumulation of the "vital essences" of the body. These are the meridians of the kidneys, liver, spleen, heart, lungs and pericardium. The other six are more yang, with functions more related to the transport of fluids and food. These are the meridians of the urinary bladder, the gall bladder, the stomach, the large intestine, the small intestine and the triple heater (the mechanism that regulates the overall temperature of the body in its upper, middle and lower parts, the Jiaos. There are also the six extraordinary meridians, one of which runs along the central and frontal line of the body: Ren Mai or Conception Vessel, and another along the spine: Du Mai or Governor Vessel.

When a TCM therapist says that an organ is out of balance, he or she is usually referring to the meridian related to that organ, not necessarily to the organ itself. For example, the liver meridian runs from the big toe, up the inside of the leg, past the genitals and into the liver itself. There can be problems along the meridians and each organ has a sphere of influence in the body. The Liver controls the free flow of general chi in the body, including emotional balance, digestion and menstruation. It also accumulates blood, regulates circulation in the tendons, has a major influence on the eyes and manifests itself in the nails. It is therefore possible to see how diseases in these areas can be treated through the Liver meridian.

In case of illness, various meridians show different disharmonic tendencies. For example, the Spleen meridian tends to a deficiency that creates "Dampness", which causes symptoms such as diarrhea or laxity (fatigue). On the other hand, the Liver tends to raise Yang, which produces red eyes, migraines and high blood pressure. Chinese medicine addresses these disharmonies.

Here are the herbs used by TCM to treat trigeminal neuralgia:

- **Gentian**

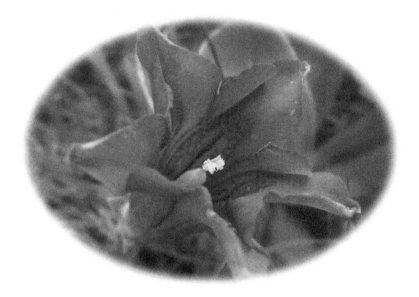

In ancient times, gentian was considered an antidote for poisonous bites, a medicine for liver and stomach problems, and a solution for cramps and fevers.

As early as the 20th century, gentian was discovered to be a powerful remedy for infectious germs.

Today, the medicinal properties of gentian include:

- **Digestive problems:** its content in bitter principles facilitates the production of digestive juices and the assimilation of enzymes, which makes it an excellent remedy against the problems of stomach, by facilitating the digestion and the defecation, by eliminating the flatulences accumulated in the stomach, by removing the feeling of heaviness, by preventing the intestinal colics, by facilitating the assimilation of food, by stimulating the appetite and by fighting muscular weakness. Its gastro-stimulating properties make it a very valuable medicinal plant in cases of: asthenia, anorexia, anemia, gastrointestinal atony, convalescence, biliary dyskinesia, gastrointestinal spasms and indigestion, among others.

- **Diuretic:** it protects the liver, purifies the blood and promotes urination, helping to eliminate toxins and reduce sodium levels. Its diuretic properties confirm that gentian is an appropriate medicinal plant for liver failure, to prevent leukopenia, kidney stones, to stop hypertension and to strengthen the immune system.

- **Dermatological problems:** the lipids contained in gentian give it a strong anti-inflammatory and healing action, very useful in case of wounds, some cases of eczema and skin spots, psoriasis and some diseases related to joints, such as gout, arthritis and rheumatism.

- **Intestinal worms:** it has vermifuge properties that make it a powerful natural vermifuge, capable of expelling intestinal worms.

- **Baldness:** its zinc content includes it in preparations that combat hair loss and the appearance of dandruff.

- Finally, its **antibiotic and antipyretic** properties give gentian the ability to reduce fever and treat bacterial diseases, such as otitis, bronchitis, flu and nasopharyngitis, among others.

Some of its constituents stimulate the production of thyroid hormones, thus contributing to the treatment of hypothyroidism.

Gentian does not generally have harmful effects, if taken in the short term. But large doses of gentian can cause vomiting, headaches or poor digestion.

The use of gentian is not recommended for pregnant or breastfeeding women, children and people with ulcers or gastritis.

It is recommended to take the mother tincture without alcohol..

- **Oriental wormwood**

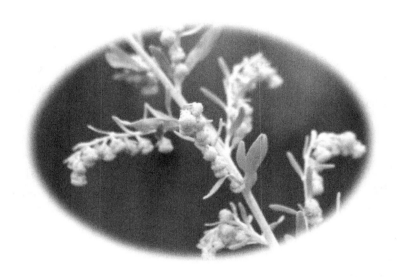

Because of its bitterness, it is very beneficial for digestive problems such as flatulence and poor digestion, as it stimulates the production of the hormone gastrin, which helps to direct food in the best way. It fights lack of appetite, because the bitter principles increase the movements of the stomach. Therefore, this plant can be given to people who are anorexic, malnourished or weakened.

Wormwood is very beneficial in the treatment of liver diseases. Thanks to its cholagogic and choleretic properties, it is very useful for this type of problem.

It has anti-inflammatory and diuretic properties, which is why it is used in the treatment of osteoarthritis and rheumatoid arthritis.

As it is diuretic, this plant is also used as a supplement for weight loss.

Due to its expectorant properties, it helps to improve respiratory problems involving mucus, such as colds, chills and flu.

There are preparations of this plant which, when applied to a painful joint, can relieve pain and reduce inflammation in cases of sprains, dislocations, tears, fractures, tendonitis, etc.

Wormwood has bactericidal, fungicidal and vulnerary properties, which makes it ideal for treating skin problems such as wounds and injuries.

The emmenagogues in this herb promote the flow of menstrual blood, so it can be used to treat certain menstrual abnormalities.

It serves as a tonic for your body, revitalizing and energizing.

You can take it in the form of infusion, tablets or capsules.

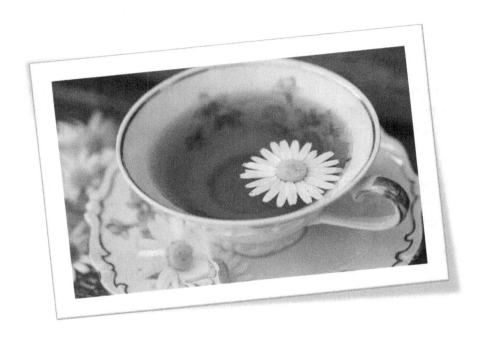

Only nature does great things without expecting anything in return.

Aromatherapy

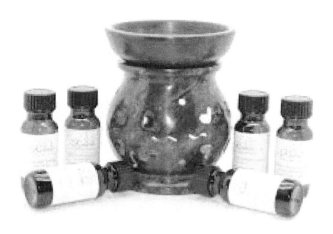

Aromatherapy is now a widely practiced complementary medicine that uses essential oils from aromatic plants, flowers, leaves, seeds, barks and fruits to aid in healing. Essential oils are usually extracted through a steam distillation process and are often used:

- Holistically, where the oils are used (often with massage) to treat emotional and physical disorders.

- Clinically, used in combination with formal medical treatments.

- Cosmetically, where they are perhaps most widely used, oils are used in burners or diffusers in the home or added to baths.

Aromatherapy works on our sense of smell and by absorption into the bloodstream. About 15% of the air we inhale reaches the nasal cavity, where olfactory receptors carry odors directly to a part of the brain called the limbic system.

It is believed that ancient civilizations used aromatherapy in many ways and for many reasons, such as massages, baths, as medicine and even to embalm bodies.

This area is linked to instinct, mood and emotion and it is believed that aromatherapy can stimulate the release of chemicals that play a role in releasing emotions (think about how even the simple smell of floor wax can quickly take you back to school days).

Aromatherapy is a careful and practical therapy that aims to induce relaxation, increase energy, reduce the effects of stress and restore the lost balance of mind, body and soul.

Robert Tisserand.

Aromatherapy seems to have its most beneficial effect on minor ailments, digestive problems, premenstrual syndrome, stress-related illnesses and certain skin problems. Some essential oils, such as tea tree, are widely used for their antiseptic properties.

Aromatherapy is unlikely to cure major illnesses, but it can be used to alleviate psychological stress in people with serious conditions such as T.N.

I have compiled **3 treatments** that aromatherapy offers us:

- Massage the affected area with eucalyptus, lavender or chamomile oil or put an infusion of these plants in the bath.

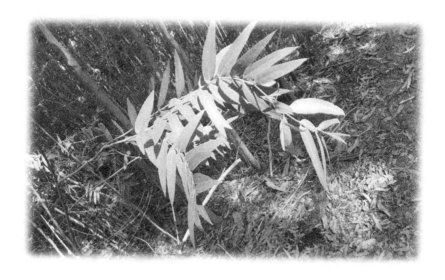

- The compress made with rosemary oil will improve circulation in the area, which will promote healing.

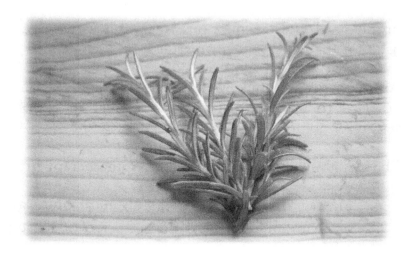

- Mix a drop of mustard and pepper oil in a little grape seed oil and massage the affected area.

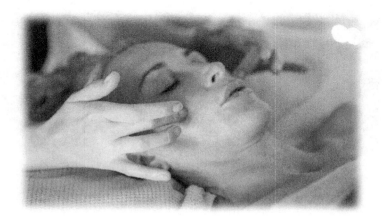

Homeopathy

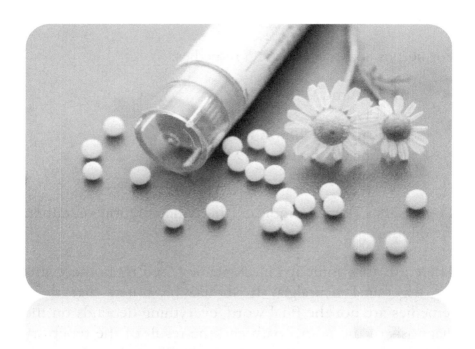

This system was created in 1810 by Dr. Hahnemann. Homeopathy is a therapeutic method that applies the phenomenon of the **law of similitude** in medical practice. It is a natural pharmacotherapy that respects in its prescription a set of basic principles and natural laws and uses micro-doses of substances from the three kingdoms (vegetable, mineral, animal) to induce a curative response.

Homeopathy treats the sick person by trying to restore the balance of his vital energy. According to the principle of similarity, the medicinal substance acts in favor of the symptom, which triggers a cellular self-healing reaction, contrary to what conventional drugs do. I advise you to be followed by a homeopath for maximum effectiveness.

For herpes zoster, there are 5 remedies:

- Mezereum D3
- Apis D3
- Rhus toxicodendron D6-10
- Ranunculus bulbosus D2-4
- Mercurius solubilis D4

The letters D or CH indicate the concentration or rather: the dilution.

There are also homeopathic remedies used by homeopaths for trigeminal neuralgia. It should be noted that these remedies are not the final word, everything depends on the diagnosis of the homeopath and the result of the repertory made by the appropriate professional. They should only be considered as a very useful aid, the rest will be left to the vital force of each person to recover.

All these remedies are readily available in pharmacies specializing in homeopathy, either prepared by accredited laboratories or prepared in the pharmacy. However, for didactic reasons, I use an almost allopathic approach for your better understanding. In any case, these formulas are not an allopathic application of homeopathy, but an application with a philosophical-homeopathic basis with the criterion of continuing the treatment with the basic medicine if the symptoms persist, are recurrent, or if they are not treated with the same medicine as the original.

- When the neuralgia occurs after a cold shock, ACONITUM NAPELLUS 6CH, twice a day, is usually recommended.
- In cases where the person feels that the pain comes in waves, and radiates during the day, KALMIA LATIFOLIA 6CH is usually recommended, also twice a day.
- When the neuralgia is on the right side, it is usual to choose MAGNESIA PHOSPHORIC 6CH, once or twice a day, depending on the intensity of the pain.
- If the neuralgia is nocturnal on the left side of the face, and especially dental neuralgia; this type of neuralgia usually comes in waves, and subsides on rising. In these cases, MAGNESIA CARBONIQUE CH. is usually used twice a day.
- In neuralgia that appears or intensifies during the menstrual period, ACTEA RACEMOSA 6CH is usually recommended, the same number of doses as above.
- When the onset is due to trauma, the first thing that is usually prescribed is ARNICA 6CH, to which you can add HYPERICUM PERFORATUM 6CH, both times a day, alternating, and as far apart as possible.
- In case of extremely acute pain, COLOCYNTHIS 6CH, 4 globules or 10 drops, can be added every 10 minutes at the time of the crisis.
- When neuralgia is accompanied by nervousness and psychic agitation, ARSENICUM ALBUM 6CH, once or twice a day, is generally recommended.

There is also a formula for nerve pain such as trigeminal neuralgia that you can ask your pharmacist.

Its composition is as follows:

Aconitum D4, Cedron D4, Colocynthis D6, Kalmia D3, Verbascum D2.

The preparation contains strong antineuralgic components.

Dosage: in case of severe crisis for ¼ to ½ hour 10 drops in a little water. For long term prevention of relapses 3 times a day 10 to 15 drops before meals in a little water.

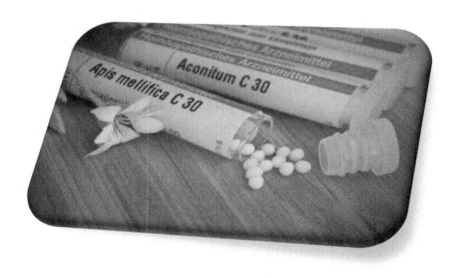

Neuromuscular Taping

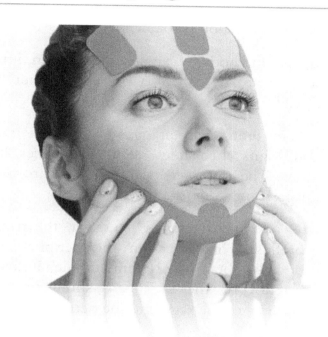

This technique has several names, Kinesio Taping, Kinesio Tape, Neurofascial Taping, Kinesiology Tape, Exteroceptive Taping... It is a taping technique born in Japan and Korea in the 70s by Dr. Kenszo Kase, Japanese chiropractor. The method allows for greater painless mobility of the musculoskeletal system thanks to bandages with a certain elasticity. It is possible to stimulate the area for several hours or days without interruption by leaving the bandages in place.

The elastic bandage is 100% cotton and uses medical cyanoacrylate as an adhesive on the opposite side. The transverse direction is totally inelastic.

With this method we can stretch, shorten, lift or drain the area we want. It can also be wet without having to be removed.

With neuromuscular taping we can treat muscles, fascia, lymph, joints, mechanics, segments, spaces, ligaments and tendons. The effects we can work on are tone, analgesia, drainage, joint support and neuroreflex.

In the case of trigeminal neuralgia, the desired effect is neuroreflex. That is, from the periphery, through the bandage, we obtain an afferent stimulus inflicted directly to the interior of the organism, stimulating the different components of the segment, the dermatome.

To be honest, this technique is perhaps the least effective of all those presented in this book. In fact, I have incorporated it in case the user would like to add it, as a co-assistant, to the combination of the other methods in order to obtain greater relief of the condition during the acute phase, but at no time has a definitive cure been observed with this treatment alone. I wanted to make available to the therapist and the patient all the methods I could find and test.

1st tape:

- ➢ first L-shaped band, 25% central stretch.
- ➢ We adhere the center just in front of the ear, in front of the temporomandibular joint (TMJ).
- ➢ Non-stretched end anchors.

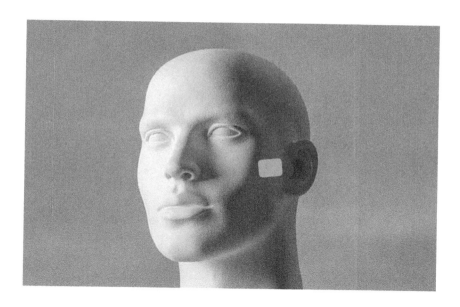

2nd tape:

> ➤ 2nd tape in an L-shape, towards the chin with the first anchor at the level of the body of the jaw, without stretching it to the end.

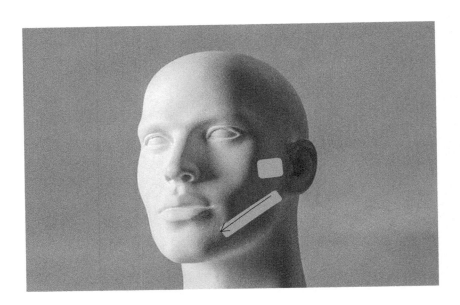

3rd tape:

> ➤ 3rd band in L-shape, towards the nose, with the 1st anchor in the maxillary region, without stretching to the end.

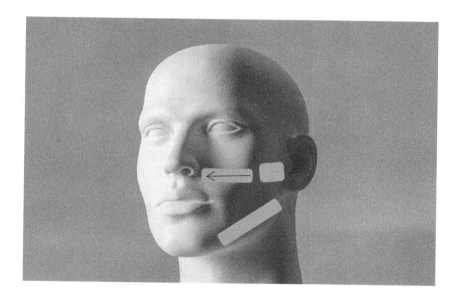

4th tape:

> ➤ 4th L band, towards the eyebrow, overlapping it, with the 1st anchor in the temporal region, without stretching along the whole length.

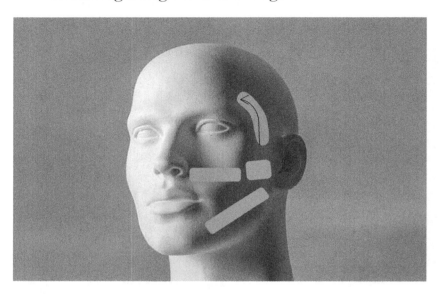

It is not necessary to apply all four tapes, you can always apply the tape n°1 and the one corresponding to the affected branch(es) of the trigeminal, whether it is the upper ophthalmic, the middle maxilla or the lower mandible.

It is important not to put too much tension on the central tape (#1) to avoid further irritating the nerve. It is also important that it covers the temporomandibular joint. The tapes of the 3 branches will always go without tension.

Classical Acupuncture

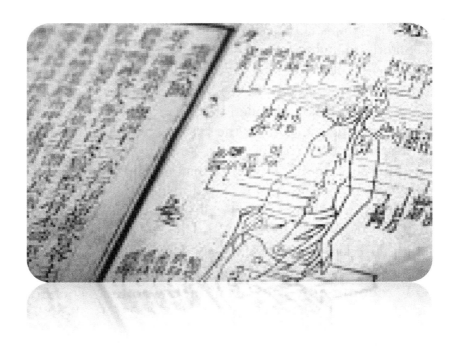

This ancient technique can be very effective for many people. In my personal experience, I must say that it was not always definitive. It works best in combination with other acupuncture techniques such as Zonal, Yamamoto or Tung acupuncture. Used as a single tool, the sessions are usually numerous and not decisive.. This therapy is exclusively for acupuncturists and includes all points that work on trigeminal neuralgia, pain, immune system, psyche, as well as herpes zoster virus.

The patient can tell the therapist to apply the acupuncture points from the list below if they wish. You can also use it if you do not want to or cannot apply Tung, Zonal or Yamamoto.

I especially recommend the points for herpes zoster that are not found in the other types of acupuncture listed. These 3 points, 22GB, 23GB and 36ST should be MUST-HITS and are highly recommended.

I have detailed below the 13 points of classical acupuncture, 10 directly treat neuralgia, heat or pain and 3 treat the virus. I have detailed the location, the technique to be used and their action on the body. The photographs are only a reminder for the therapist.

Classical acupuncture indicates that certain points can be subjected to moxibustion. Moxibustion is one of the therapeutic techniques of Traditional Chinese Medicine (TCM) in which pure Moxa (made from the mugwort plant) is used to apply heat to specific acupuncture points and increase the benefits of treatment. Personally, **I do NOT recommend moxa on facial points**. Therefore, only 3LI, 36ST, 3LI, 62UB, 22GB and 23GB should be moxied.

The person who is not at peace with himself is at war with the whole world.

Ghandi

7 ST – Sia Kuan

Location: closed mouth, in the depression formed between the zygomatic arch and the mandibular incisure.

Technique: 0.3 - 0.5 Tsun perpendicular + moxibustion.

Action : disperses wind and releases heat, soothes pain and sharpens hearing.

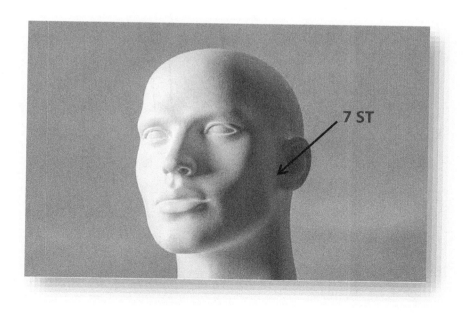

3 LI – Sann Tsienn

<u>Location</u>: with the hand relaxed, in the proximal and radial depression of the 2nd metacarpophalangeal joint.

<u>Technique</u>: 0.3 - 0.5 Tsun perpendicular + moxibustion.

<u>Action</u>: clears heat and eliminates acute inflammations of the head, face, eyes, mouth and ENT area.

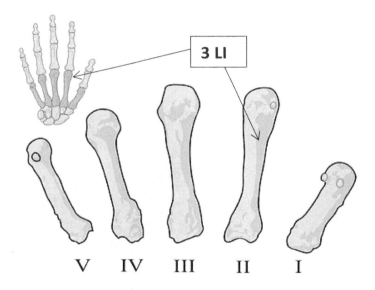

3 LI

V   IV   III   II   I

If the essential energy of man is balanced
other pathogenic energies will not be able to attack him.

Nguyen Van Nghi

4 ST – Ti Tsang

Location: looking straight ahead, under the pupil, 0.4 Tsun laterally towards the corner of the mouth.

Technique: 0.2 Tsun perpendicular or 0.5 - 0.8 Tsun subcutaneously towards E6 + moxibustion.

Action : Dispersing the wind and making the ramifications practicable.

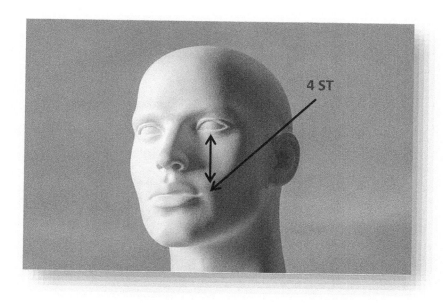

36 ST – San Li

<u>Location</u>: Knee flexed, 3 Tsun under the depression of the lower border of the patella, laterally towards the anterior tibial border, at the level of the distal border of the anterior tibial tuberosity.

<u>Technique</u>: 1-2 perpendicular Tsun + moxibustion.

<u>Action</u> : Important point against the virus. Strengthens the body, reinforces the Spleen, harmonizes the Stomach, regulates and balances the energetic mechanism, decongests the meridian and its branches and makes them practicable. Strengthens immunity.

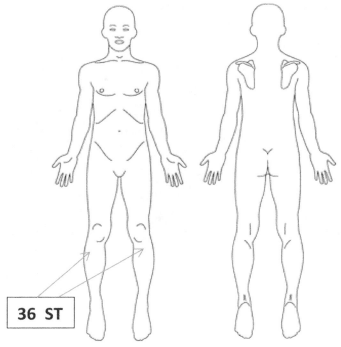

36 ST

3 LI – Jeou Tsi

<u>Location</u>: the fist slightly clenched, at the ulnar end of the proximal transverse fold, at the level of the 5th metacarpophalangeal joint, at the limit between the red and white flesh.

<u>Technique</u>: 0.3 - 0.5 Tsun perpendicular + moxibustion

<u>Action</u> : Clears the heart and provides general sedation, eliminates inflammation, increases visual acuity. Helps psychic and psychosomatic disorders.

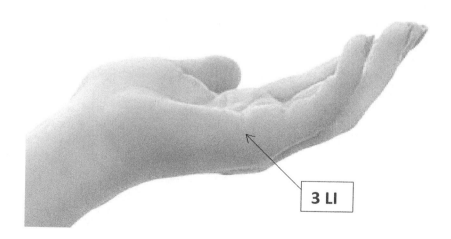

3 LI

18 LI – Tsiuann Tsiao

Location: Right, under the external corner of the eye, in the lower depression of the zygomatic arch.

Technique: 0.3 - 0.5 Tsun perpendicular + moxibustion.

Action : Soothes pain and acts in particular on trigeminal neuralgia.

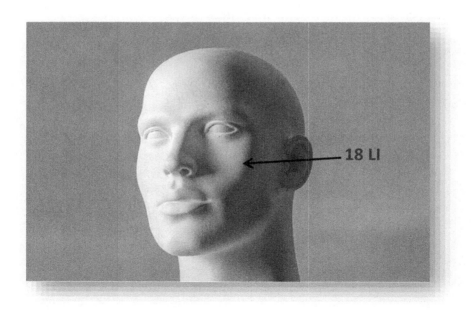

19 LI – Ting King

Location: half-open mouth, in the anterior depression of the tragus and behind the mandibular head.

Technique: 1 - 1.05 Tsun perpendicular + moxibustion

Action : Acts on trigeminal neuralgia (especially the 1st branch)

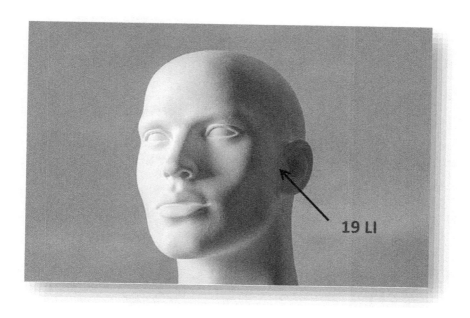

62 UB – Chen Mo

Location: In the distal depression of the lateral malleolus.

Technique: 0.3 - 0.5 Tsun perpendicular + moxibustion.

Action : Headaches, dizziness and stupor. Sleep disorders, epilepsy, psychic and psychosomatic disorders (sedative and antispasmodic action).

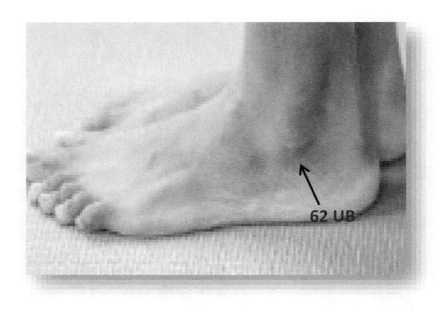

Energy is the cause of all production and destruction.

Nei King Su Wen

21 TH – El Menn

Location: In front of the superior incision of the tragus, in the craniodorsal depression of the condyle of the mandible.

Technique: 0.5 - 1 Tsun perpendicular + moxibustion.

Action : specific trigeminal neuralgia. Makes the meridian practicable.

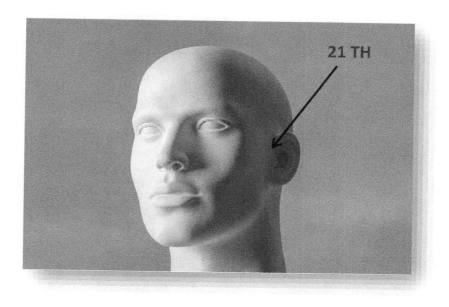

2 GB – Ting Joe

<u>Location</u>: open mouth, in front of the intertragal incisure, in the dorsal depression of the mandibular condyle.

<u>Technique</u>: 0.5 - 1 Tsun perpendicular + moxibustion.

<u>Action</u> : Ear diseases and trigeminal neuralgia.

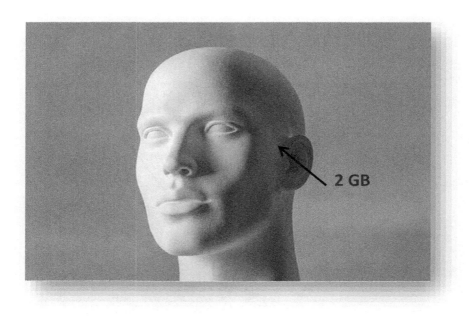

Some claim, including myself, that we do not have a skeleton, muscles, glands, nervous system but that "we are all of these".

Moshé Feldenkrais

22 GB – Luann lé

Location: raised arm, in the mid-axillary line, 3 Tsun below the armpit, in the 4th intercostal space.

Technique: 0.5 - 0.8 Tsun oblique or subcutaneous + moxibustion.

Action : soothes pain, specific against herpes zoster.

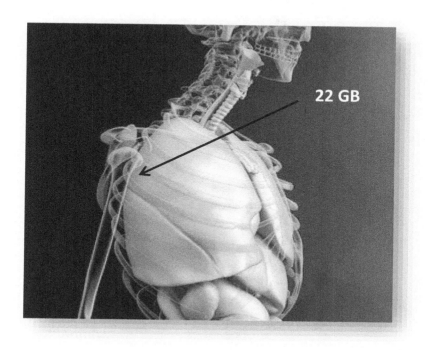

23 GB – Tché

<u>Location</u>: 1 Tsun in front of GB 22, in the 4th intercostal space, at the level of the nipple.

<u>Technique</u> : 0,5 - 0,8 Tsun oblique or subcutaneous + moxibustion.

<u>Action</u> : It puts order in the energy and calms the pain. Specific against herpes zoster.

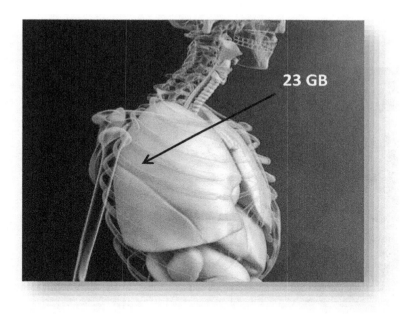

When man is removed from nature, he gradually loses his health.

Manuel Lezaeta

Secondary point of the head and neck 5 - Traé Yang

<u>Location</u>: In the depression between the outer edge of the eyebrow and the outer corner of the eye.

<u>Technique</u>: 0.3 - 0.5 Tsun perpendicular or oblique + micro-needling.

<u>Action</u>: releases heat, soothes pain and relaxes the branches. Trigeminal neuralgia.

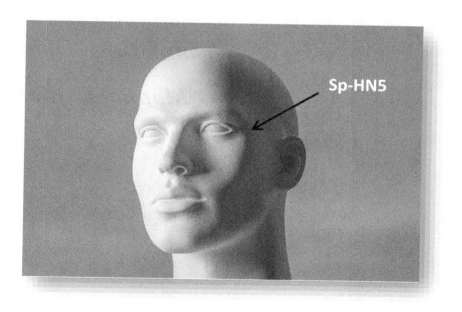

Four things must be eliminated at the beginning: debts, fire, enemies and diseases.

Confucius

When the human body is cut off from nature, it gradually loses its health.

Manuel Lezaeta

Auriculothérapie Chinoise

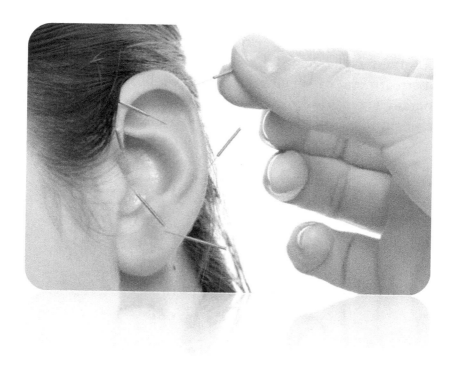

Auriculotherapy is also known as **Auriculopuncture**. It is a technique that comes from acupuncture. It consists of stimulating certain points that exist in the ear.

Traditional Chinese medicine uses the energy meridians to treat various ailments, by seeking a balance of energies. What we call energy is nothing more than the electrical impulses that circulate in our body.

Auriculopuncture is based on the fact that in the ear is a representation of all parts of our body. Thus, any pathology or ailment can be treated from the ear, by stimulating specific points on the external auditory pinna. You can use short needles, a laser, micro-magnets, quartz or pins for auriculotherapy and even specific seeds for this therapy. I recommend the use of an electronic point detector if possible, it will help you identify them accurately and rule out those that do not need to be stimulated. It is recommended to leave the needles on for 15-30 minutes. The treatment of trigeminal neuralgia by auriculotherapy generally gives good results, even if it often happens that at the beginning, a curative phase appears, i.e. a worsening of the symptoms for a few days to then give way to an improvement.

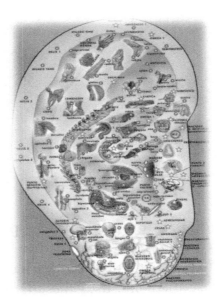

When the mind is calm and stable, the vitality of life circulates harmoniously throughout the body. If the body is nourished and protected by the circulating vitality, how is it possible to become ill?

Classical internal medicine of the Yellow Emperor (2nd century BC)

Let's define the main parts of the external ear.

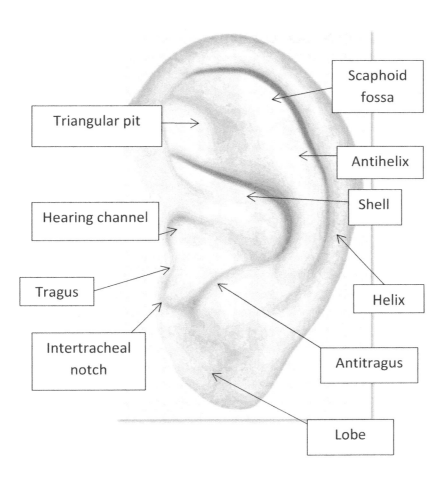

Auriculotherapy, also known as **auricular medicine**, is an age-old technique recognized and approved by the World Health Organization (WHO) since 1990. It is used not only for the diagnosis and treatment of pain, but also for addictions, internal disorders and basic emotional problems.

Contraindications

Frostbite, injuries, clotting problems, heart problems or severe anemia, during menstruation at specific times and for pregnant women.

Points to treat :

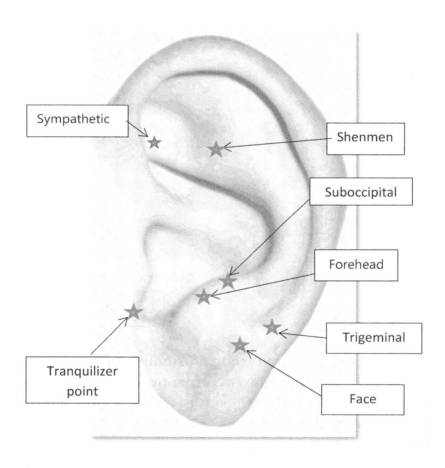

Osteopathy

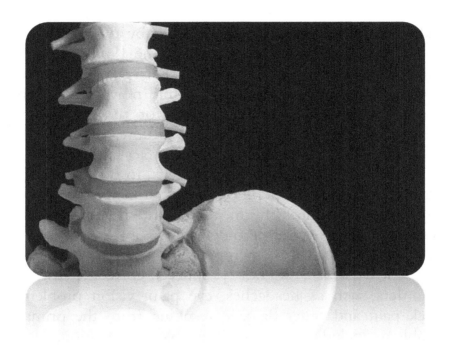

My years of experience have shown me that this disease is more biochemical than physical. I have no doubt that if we alleviate a certain affected area, it can contribute to an improvement and help the pain disappear, but it clearly does not result in the total eradication of the condition. However, I will indicate what can be done on a physical level with osteopathy. Of course, these techniques are for osteopathic professionals and cannot be used by the patient himself.

The first step that the osteopath must employ is the release of the fascias. These first two exercises will effectively release the fascias but it is at the same time a cranial osteopathic treatment. These first two osteopathic techniques focus on the primary respiratory movement that begins in the 5th month of uterine life. This respiratory movement, called primary because it begins before pulmonary respiration at birth, is caused by the pumping of the cerebrospinal fluid contained in the skull and dural tube, which runs along the spine. This pumping, which produces a similar slow and rhythmic movement in the tissues, must exist and be correct, for the central and peripheral nervous system to be healthy, and for the movements of the cranial bones, the face and the entire spine, including the sacrum and coccyx, to be able to take place correctly. In addition, this primary respiratory movement influences the movement of the fascia in the rest of the body. With sacro-cranial osteopathy, the goal is to recover optimal CSF pumping and primary respiratory movement which, if not produced correctly, triggers disorders such as headaches, eye pain, vision problems, back pain and other damage resulting from the primary problem, including emotional problems, agitation, sleep problems, etc...I will not go into detail in the description, as all osteopaths are very familiar with these techniques. A complete work would consist in relaxing the fascias (connective tissue) of the neck, then readjusting the cervical vertebrae, especially C3, and finishing with a cranial osteopathic treatment to work on the cranial nerves.

Occipital pumping.

With this rhythmic decompression work, we will have a cranio-sacral effect on the whole connective tissue and a relaxation of the deep muscles. This exercise is indicated in vertebral pathologies, neurological pathologies and in cases of emotional tension.

Realization of the technique: _the patient is in a lying position. The osteopath is in a sitting position, at the head of the table. The technique consists in holding the occipital of the patient with both hands and pumping, at a rate of 3 seconds of traction and 3 seconds of semi-relaxation, during 1 to 3 minutes._

We will let the occipital protuberances rest on the tips of the fingers which will have a direction towards the orbits. The nape of the neck will sink little by little on the fingers, the muscles will give way and relax. The osteopath will be able to reach the posterior arch of the atlas and then exercise light traction and relaxation.

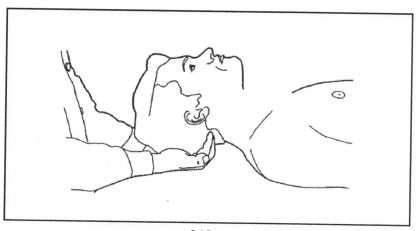

Sacrum pumping.

Execution of the technique: The patient is in the supine or back position (I recommend the back position). The osteopath stands on one side of the patient. With the caudal hand, we contact the sacrum of the patient, fixing the abdomen of the patient with the cranial hand. The technique consists in carrying out, with the caudal hand, a rhythmic pumping of the sacrum at a rate of 3 seconds of traction and 3 seconds of semi-relaxation, during 1 to 3 minutes

This exercise is indicated in spinal pathologies, in neurological pathologies and in cases of emotional tension.

The following figure shows the exercise with the patient in pronation.

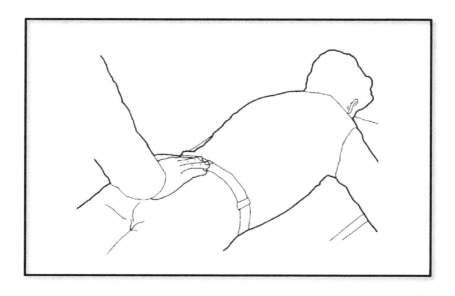

The main function of this technique is to correct imbalances or dysfunctions that may exist in the spine, limbs and any organic area.
Over time, the body adapts to these imbalances and specific characteristics appear.

The fingers that think, feel and see are our instrument. They feel and see how the tissue moves, this art is known as osteopathy.

Dr. William Garner Sutherland

Osteopathy tells us that sometimes, due to muscle dysfunction, a trapping of the 5th cranial nerve can occur at a certain point in the pathway. These naturopathies can lead to a change in the conductivity of the nerve impulses.

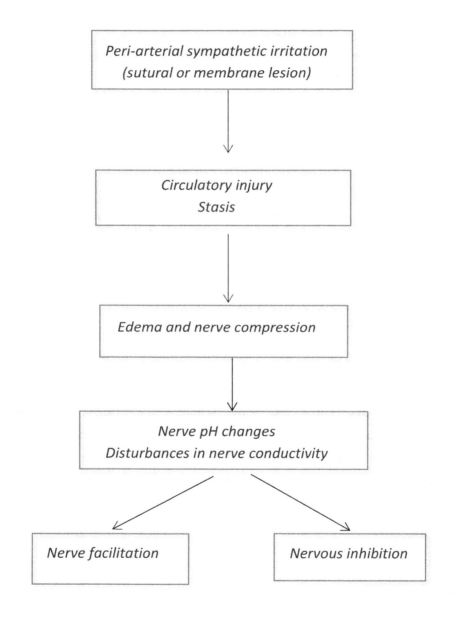

In order to free the 3 trigeminal branches, it is essential that the large wing of the sphenoid be free of any dysfunction; it is also necessary to check the relationships at this level:

- Fronto-sphenoidal

- Parietal-sphenoidal

- Spheno-temporal

- Spheno-maxillary

- Sphenopetal

The trigeminal nerve is one of the cranial nerves that forces the osteopath to free up practically the entire cranial sphere.

Cerebrospinal fluid fluctuates rhythmically within a natural cavity: the neurocranium, and can be observed by our palpation. It is because the body is fundamentally composed of fluids and this cerebrospinal fluid is partly absorbed by the lymphatic system, that we can observe the fluctuation of cerebrospinal fluid throughout the body.

Dr. Rollin E. Becker

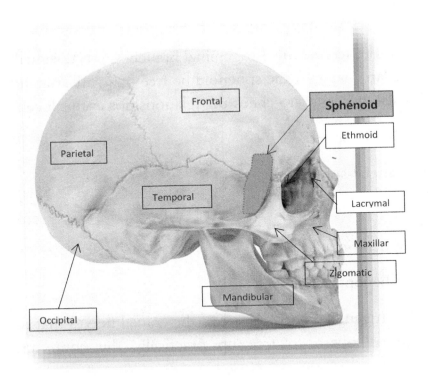

Finding health should be the goal of the therapist,
anyone can find illness.

Dr. Andrew Taylor Still

Finally, we recommend an evaluation and rectification if necessary of the cervical spine, particularly focused on the third cervical (C3).

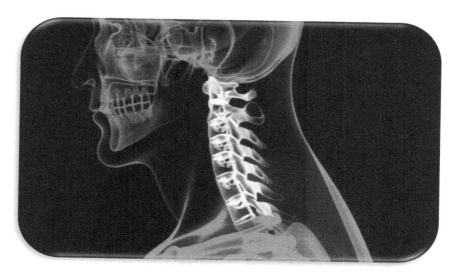

Although trigeminal neuralgia as a presentation of cervical pathology is rare in studies to date, it should be considered a differential diagnosis. The anatomic-pathologic explanation lies in the fact that the trigeminal spinal nucleus terminates in the cervical segments of C2 to C3 and that nociceptive impulses from the neck can synapse there and trigger a picture of this type.

As we do not want to forget anything in the treatment of this terrible pathology, we can look for a good osteopath to release the fascias, adjust the CSF impulse along the spine, check the relationships of the cranial bones and adjust the cervical spine. If this work is not satisfactory at the level of our pain, I can assure you that it will be satisfactory at other levels that you will quickly notice.

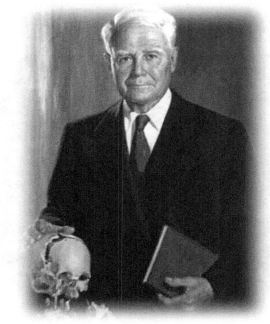

William Sutherland

(Iconic figure in American osteopathic medicine)

Combien d'entre nous souhaitent être soulagés de leurs problèmes, mais n'ont pas la moindre idée de changer leurs précieuses façons de vivre, de sentir, de penser et de croire...

Dr. Viola Frymann

Yamamoto Craniopuncture

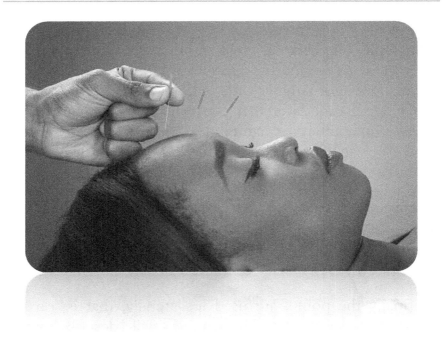

Yamamoto Craniopuncture is a comprehensive system of acupuncture assessment, diagnosis and treatment developed by Japanese physician Toshikatsu Yamamoto. Yamamoto's craniopuncture began to be researched in the 1960s and was presented in 1973 at the Ryodoraku Congress in Osaka. Throughout this period until today (more than 40 years), Dr. Yamamoto has continued to research and improve the system: he has discovered many more points, not only in the head, but also in other parts of the body.

Yamamoto's cranial acupuncture method is the most widely used microsystem in the world after Auriculopuncture. It is considered to be a very effective system in the treatment of acute and chronic pain, in the treatment of many neurological disorders and in an infinite number of pathologies. I have a great fondness for this therapy because of its wonderful results and ease of application. If the reader is not familiar with acupuncture needles, you can use a therapeutic laser that you can buy in various online sales of equipment for natural therapies. If you can't find it, send me an email so I can help you, if you wish. Yamamoto's technique works perfectly with the laser, unlike zonal acupuncture, for example. It also gives faster results than traditional acupuncture. When the acupuncturist reaches the desired point, there may be a kind of small electrical discharge or pain, Chinese medicine describes this as Qi.

Normally the points are used ipsilaterally, that is, on the same part of the assignment. I will describe when contralateral application is recommended.

To perform the puncture of the needle, we will introduce it with an angle of about 15°, that is, its insertion will be almost horizontal to the skin and the whole needle should be introduced (about 2 cm). The type of needle is not important. The number of sessions varies from one individual to another, so there is no fixed amount, as in almost all alternative therapies.

The time during which the needles must remain in place will be about 20 to 30 minutes in acute cases and even one hour in chronic phases. This treatment can also be combined with electro-acupuncture, adjusting the frequency between 5 and 15 Hz and applying it with an intensity that is not unpleasant for the patient. Personally, I never treat trigeminal neuralgia with electricity because the patient is tired of the shocks produced by the pathology. If laser acupuncture is used, about 5 minutes per point is sufficient, also depending on the intensity of the device. I have been able to verify that Yamamoto acupuncture combined with zonal acupuncture gives quick and effective results.

Basically, this therapy is based on acupuncture points established mainly on the skull and exclusively in the case of trigeminal neuralgia. The system gives excellent results as a single therapy, especially in conjunction with the others. It is a totally painless system, both in terms of the needles and the laser.

I do not intend with this book to give a course in acupuncture, there are already many on the market, I will only focus on teaching the reader to locate the points that really work in the treatment of trigeminal neuralgia and how to apply the needles or the laser.

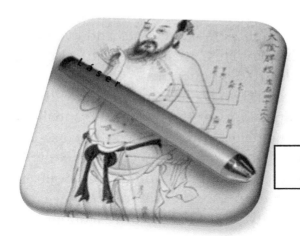

Laser acupuncture

In acupuncture as in laser-puncture, when you look for the point, you must look for a painful point very close to this point. That is to say, you have to feel with a finger a little bit around the place where the point is and puncture at this more sensitive place. If you are using a laser, the device itself can be used to find the sore spot by pressing a little on the area instead of using your finger, if you prefer. It is very important to look for these ASHI points, or tender points.

POINT 1

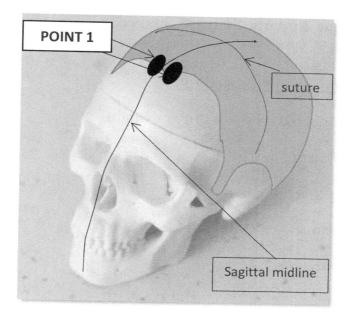

Point 1 is located about 1 cm lateral to the sagittal midline, on the hairline or about 5-6 cm anterior to the coronal suture. This point is approximately 2 cm long, has a portion below the hairline (1 cm) and a portion above the hairline (1 cm). If the patient has no hair, we will ask him/her to frown (muscle contraction of the forehead and between the eyebrows) and we will then take the upper forehead wrinkle as a reference.

This point is particularly recommended for **trigeminal neuralgia**.

This point is also indicated for:

- Headaches and migraines of any origin.

- Cervical pain.

- Cervico-brachialgia.

- Neuropathies.

- Facial paralysis.

- Dental pain.

- Vertigo.

- Central nervous system disorders.

- Post-stroke sequelae.

The natural force within each of us is the greatest healer of all.

Hippocrates

POINT 2

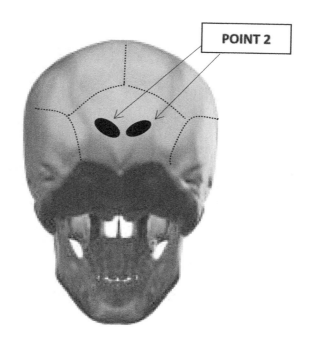

POINT 2

Located about 2 cm from the sagittal midline, in the occipital bone, forming an angle of approximately 40° and a length of about 2 cm.

In this case, it is recommended to combat the effects of herpes zoster.

This point is also indicated for :

- Pain in the chest area.
- Affections of the thoracic spine and ribs.
- Intercostal neuralgia.
- Fractures.
- Pathologies of the thoracic organs.

POINT 3

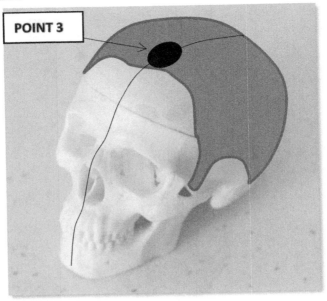

This point, which is actually a set of points called brain points, has three points: the brain, the cerebellum and the basal ganglia. In order not to complicate things too much, we will see it as a single large point but we will have to palpate it to find the area to be treated. This area of points is located with its center on the sagittal line between 4 and 5 cm long, just above point 1.

In case of acute trigeminal neuralgia, one should not puncture on the same side as the pain until the chronic phase has passed. It is interesting to know that the cranial trigeminal nerve point V passes through this point.

This point and point 1 are very effective.

This point is also appropriate for:

- Neurological pathologies.
- Motor disorders.
- Hemiplegia and paraplegia.
- Parkinson's disease.
- Endocrine disorders.
- Vertigo.
- Visual disorders.
- Tinnitus.
- aphasia
- Dementia
- Alzheimer's disease.
- Epilepsy.
- Insomnia.
- Depression.

If a person wants to be healthy, they must first ask themselves if they are ready to eliminate the reasons for their illness. Only then is it possible to help them.

Hippocrates

POINT 4

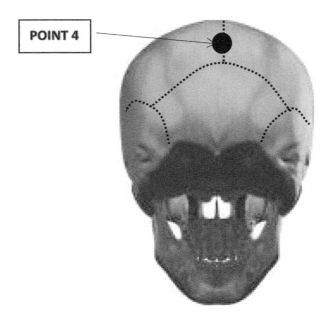

Point 4 has the same characteristics as point 3. It is in fact point 3 but further back. Its indications are exactly the same as those of point 3.

Yamamoto's craniopuncture is more complex and extensive, I wanted to simplify it to these 4 main points. As a general rule, by using only points 1 and 3, the result should be noticeable. I invite the reader to start with these two points, if they are not sufficient, he can extend it with the other two points.

Zonal Acupuncture

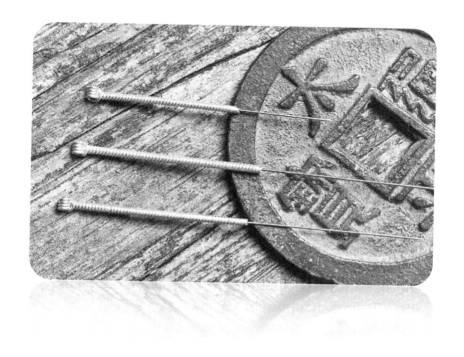

Zonal acupuncture is a technique that was discovered in the 1970s. In fact, its original name is **acupuncture of the wrist and ankle** and its inventor was Dr. Xin Zhu Zang. Josep Carrión was the main Spanish disseminator of this technique. It is a simple and very effective method that I recommend without any doubt. This little known acupuncture has nothing to do with the acupuncture meridians, it is an intradermal, superficial and subcutaneous application of needles.

I must admit that even using it solely and exclusively as a treatment for trigeminal neuralgia, the results are noticeable within a few days. It is amazing how powerful and simple this technique is.

Another important point about Zonal Acupuncture is that it is one hundred percent painless and quick to apply. In my experience, the results have even surpassed traditional acupuncture on many occasions. Its effect is often felt immediately after the needle is inserted. Technicians who discover it often do not use any other type of acupuncture afterwards. My intention in this book is not to explain all the methodology and technique of zonal acupuncture, that is not the objective, but to explain the protocol for the pathology that concerns us. I will therefore focus on explaining to the therapist where and how to insert the needle. I sincerely believe that even a non-therapist, i.e. the patient himself, with a little skill, can heal himself. If this is not the case, the person concerned can, with the help of this book, show the method to an acupuncturist so that he/she can apply acupuncture.

It is extremely important to locate the points perfectly, because an error in location will completely cancel out the desired effect.

In the case of trigeminal neuralgia, if the patient is in the acute phase, we will try to leave the needles in for a short time, at the beginning, i.e. about 15 minutes, extending the following sessions up to 45 minutes if it is well tolerated. The puncture should be done only on the affected side and in both arms if it is both cheeks.

Method:

We will use needles that are approximately 4 or 5 cm long and 0.25 to 0.30 thick.

We perform an asepsis of the area with alcohol or a topical antiseptic.

We locate the spot. If a blood vessel coincides with the point, we move slightly distally but in the same longitudinal line.

The insertion will be in the cranial direction, i.e. upwards.

The needle puncture will be placed at 30° on the skin, forming this angle with the hand, as in the following picture:

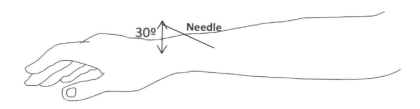

The skin is slightly pierced, pulling the needle out until it comes loose (without pulling it out of the skin) on the skin. This means that the insertion is very superficial.

We must insert at least 4 cm. It is essential that the insertion is completely painless. It must be withdrawn slightly and put back in place if any pain appears.

The needle must not be touched after insertion.

Sessions of 30 to 60 minutes, 3 times a week, are acceptable.

With this therapy, what we regulate, as with Yamamoto, is the energy part of the body. It does not always work alone, but it is indispensable, especially in the acute phases.

It consists in puncturing **3 points on the wrist, point 1 being the most important** and the following ones being complementary. Personally, I have only used point 1 and it has given me excellent results.

I will detail the exact location of the **3 points** as follows:

-Point 1-

It is located midway along the distal border of the forearm, just between the ulna and the tendon of the flexor-carpi-ulnaris muscle. At a distance of 2 inches from the wrist crease. When searching for the point, the palm of the hand should be turned towards the patient, i.e. supinated and the arm extended.

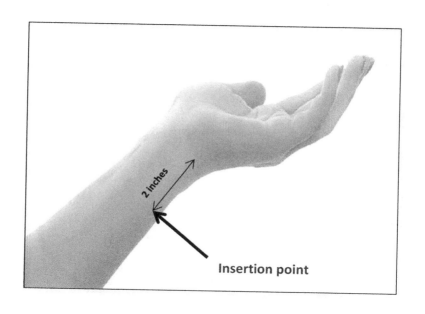

We are very interested in this point not only because it acts on the face, relieving neuralgia attacks, but also because it has been proven to help insomnia and it is well known that in many cases the patient with neuralgia has his sleep affected, as was my case.

For your information, this point n°1 is also effective for :

- frontal headaches

- ocular pathology

- nasal and facial pathology

- cardiac pathology

- gastric pathology

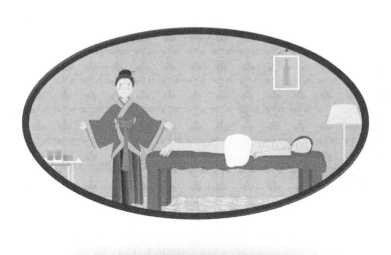

-Point 2-

It is located between the tendon of the palmaris major muscle and the flexor carpi radialis. It is found with the palm supinated and the patient is asked to clench the fist, as in the photo, to mark the tendons. The distance from the wrist crease is 2 inches. Try to avoid punctuating the blood vessels.

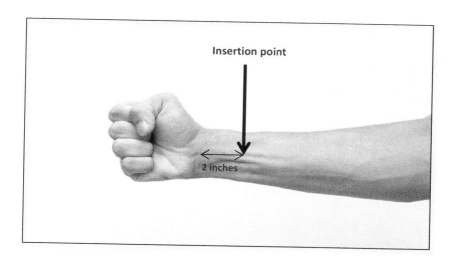

This point has a more secondary impact since it treats more the lateral zone, i.e. it covers the frontal part in its lateral margins, the temples, the cheeks, the molars and the submaxillary zone.

- For your information, this point n°2 is also effective in the following cases
- Anterotemporal headache
- Posterior odontalgia
- Breast pain and distension
- Chest pain
- Asthma
- Pneumonia

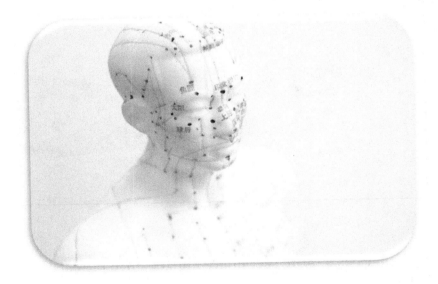

-Point 3-

This last point is located on the radial side of the radial artery, just between the radius and the radial artery. About 1cm from the radius to the artery. It should be located with the forearm in supination. It is 2 inches away from the wrist crease.

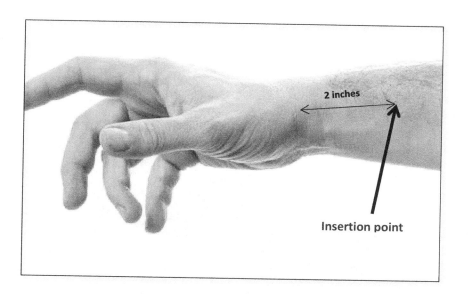

This point concerns the auricle area and the temporomandibular joint. I only recommend this point if the previous two are ineffective or as the sole treatment for trigeminal neuralgia. Of course, none of them does any harm and can be treated perfectly and all together.

For your information, this point n°3 is also effective in the following cases :

- Temporo-auricular headache

- Pain on the inside of the shoulder

- Costal pain

- Epicondylitis

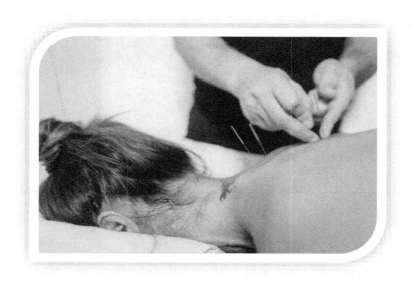

The human being spends the first half of his life ruining his health and the other half trying to restore it.

Joseph Leonard

Biomagnetic Pair

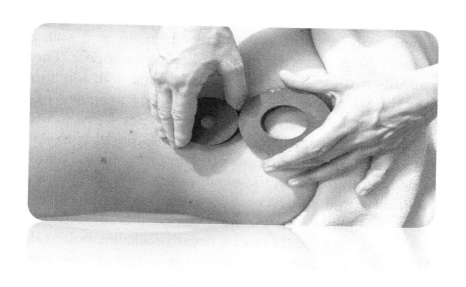

The power of magnets has been known since time immemorial, it was used by the Chinese with the invention of the compass, then by the Egyptians who crushed ferrite which they added to food to improve health. Other ancient cultures also used magnets, such as the Hindus, Arabs, Persians, Hebrews or Romans. They were used by Cleopatra, Aristotle, Pliny the Elder or Galen. Paracelsus discovered the healing effects of magnetic polarities in living beings and claimed that the Earth itself was like a great magnet. The French Royal Society of Medicine certified in 1777 the positive effects of magnetic treatments on health. The Nobel Prize winner Linus Pauling discovered the magnetic properties of hemoglobin in blood.

The largest hospitals already use all kinds of devices that work with magnets induced by an electric current creating magnetic fields as therapy.

The famous Dr. Goiz discovered and proved that it was possible to alkalize the pH of the body, thanks to a pair of magnets with opposite poles. Indeed, in an acid soil, all kinds of viruses, bacteria, fungi and parasites appear. These organisms do not survive in more alkaline soil. Dr. Goiz was right when he said that by applying magnets of a certain strength, one in North or negative polarity and the other in South or positive polarity, it was possible to level the pH, balancing the pathogen support medium until it was neutral. In this way, these pathogens cease to have vital conditions for them. A healthy tissue has a pH close to neutral (7), the pH of some areas can be altered, generating a positive acidic pole (H+) or a negative alkaline pole (OH-). When homeostasis is disrupted, one area of the body becomes acidic and another area becomes alkaline. The pH of the body should be slightly alkaline (7.3). The two poles (acid and alkaline) of a biomagnetic couple create a magnetic field inside the body and favor the development of pathogens. If the pH neutrality of the affected area is restored, the pathogen or organic dysfunction loses the environment it needs, thus restoring health.

The advantage of this technique is that the patient can apply the treatment without being aware of it, although this is always recommended. All that is needed to begin the treatment is at least one pair of strong magnets, which are easily available in stores. I recommend neodymium magnets of 12,000 Gauss and lined with leather. They are easily found on the Internet for about 10 euros each. In the following picture you can see what they look like.

**North Pole
or Negative
Black**

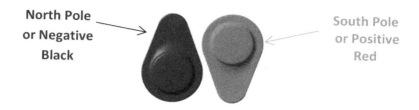

South Pole
or Positive
Red

Ideally, a specialized therapist should do what is called a kinesiology tracing to find the areas of the body to be treated. If the patient does not have one available, he or she can easily use the points I will outline below.

You will need to identify the north and south poles. Normally, the North or negative pole is black and the South or positive pole is red. I will detail the properties of each pole as follows.

<u>**North or negative pole (black)**</u>

- Reduces pain and inflammation.

- Cancels the pathogenicity of microorganisms.

- Stops the growth of certain types of tumors.

- Reduces hyperacidity.

- Reduces infections.

- Acts as a relaxant

South Pole or Positive (red)

- Increases pain and inflammation.

- Promotes the growth of microorganisms.

- Increases acidity.

- Increases energy.

- Increases the size of tumors.

- It is indicated in the cases of muscular weaknesses and muscular tears, bone and ligament fractures, sprains, in fractures of bones and ligaments, sprains, in rehabilitation, healing.

If the positive polarity of a magnet is placed in the acidic focus and the negative polarity in the alkaline area of the same pair, the H+ ions and OH- ions will be displaced and neutralize each other. The electric charge cancels out and the pH of these two foci balances as two charges of the same sign repel each other. Magnets do not heal, but they do allow the body to regain its health.

The reader will appreciate the usefulness of these magnets, and not only in their use for trigeminal neuralgia. It is easy to use and can be applied two or three times a week and 30 minutes will be sufficient. To use it as a monotherapy, the patient should choose to seek out a biomagnetic therapist who is able to trace the entire body and after several sessions eliminate the herpes zoster virus and the bacteria that support it.

It is important to know the order of magnet placement, and this depends on which hemisphere you are in. In the northern hemisphere, the negative poles of the biomagnetic pairs tend to be established in the right hemisphere. In the southern hemisphere, it is common for the negative poles to be established in the left hemisphere. In other words, in Europe or USA, the first pair (which is usually positive or red) will always be placed on the left side of the body and the second pair (which is usually negative or black) will be placed on the right side. In South America, for example, they will be applied in reverse.

Caution:

- Do not place magnets if the patient is pregnant.

- Do not place magnets within 20 cm of a pacemaker, other electronic device, or a brain valve made of ferromagnetic material.

- Do not treat a patient who has received chemotherapy within the last 12 months

or who will be receiving chemotherapy in the near future.

Ear - Ear

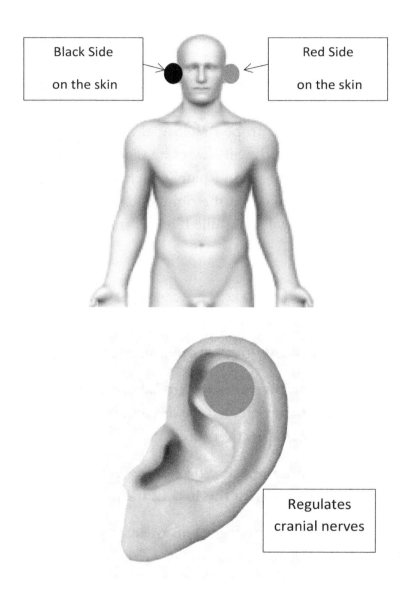

Black Side

on the skin

Red Side

on the skin

Regulates
cranial nerves

Cubitus - Cubitus

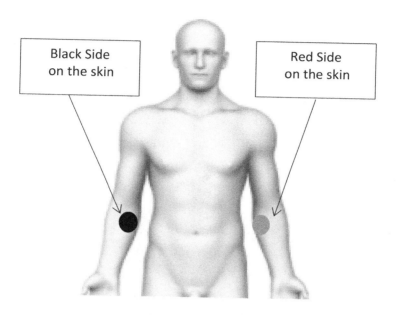

Black Side
on the skin

Red Side
on the skin

Acts on the herpes virus

Thymus – Thymus

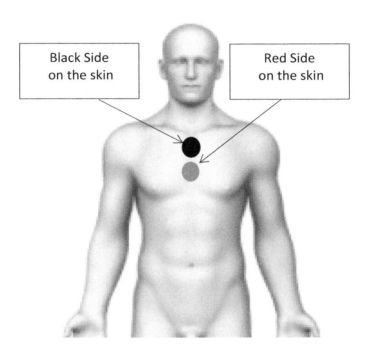

Black Side on the skin

Red Side on the skin

Increases the

immune system

Bladder - Bladder

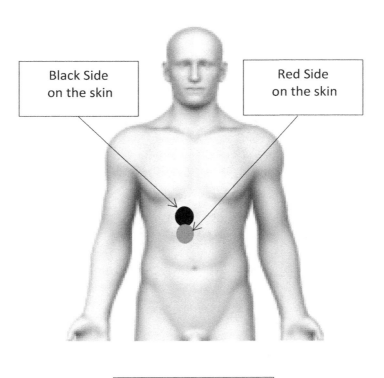

Black Side
on the skin

Red Side
on the skin

Virus reservoir

Frontal sinus - Frontal sinus

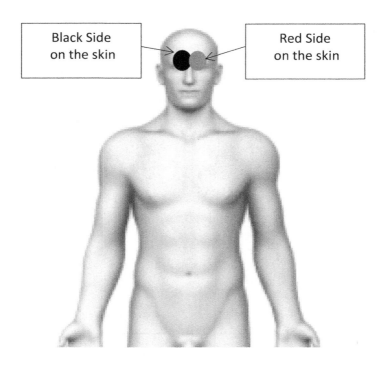

Black Side
on the skin

Red Side
on the skin

Acts on the virus

Acupuncture Tung

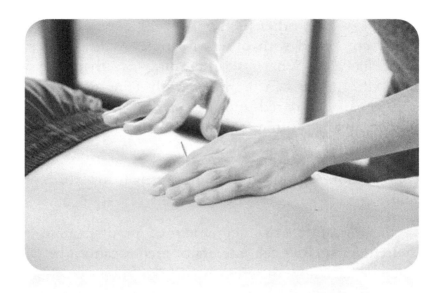

Tung acupuncture is probably one of the most mysterious and effective of all acupuncture techniques. It became known in the 1970s thanks to Dr. Jing Chan Tung, known as Master Tung. This secret technique comes from a long lineage that took refuge in Taiwan. During this decade, Master Tung allowed the partial diffusion of this art to 73 disciples. Tung's acupuncture breaks the rules of traditional acupuncture by not following the rules of the meridians and by having twice as many points. Dr. Tung took the secret of his success to his grave, but the points collected remain for the benefit of mankind. This technique does not contain many points that improve trigeminal neuralgia, but I will present here the few existing points so that the reader can incorporate them into his therapy with a high degree of effectiveness. Like other methods, in my experience, Tung must be combined with others to increase its chances of overall success. What is interesting is that classical acupuncture points can be mixed with Tung acupuncture. Diseases can be cured in one session, unlike classical acupuncture which often requires many treatments.

The needles to be used give the best results with a thickness of 0.30 mm, although I usually use 0.25 mm needles.

For the location of acupuncture points, units of measurement such as centimeters or inches cannot be used, as there are many differences in size between human beings. Therefore, anatomical references (bones, tendons) and proportional measurements or cun are used.

It is taken as a reference that 1 cun is the width of the big finger of the patient's hand.

I will detail below the 7 points that are known to affect Trigeminal Neuralgia. The 7 points are distributed in 3 different areas.

If you are not an acupuncturist, you can use a therapeutic laser on the points. The time required will be from 2 to 10 minutes, depending on the power of the laser.

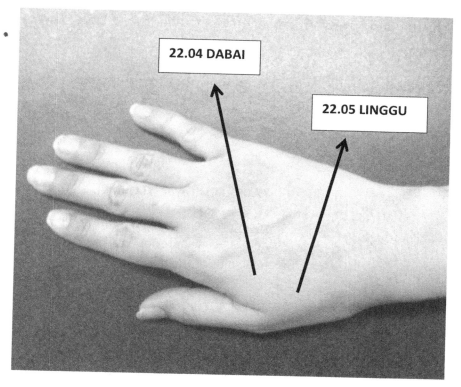

The Ling Gu point is located at the top of the hand, between the first and the second metacarpus, that is to say between the thumb and the index finger, a little above the soft area which allows the finger "alone" to articulate. If we place a finger of the other hand on this point, we will notice that there is a kind of hollow.

The Dabai point is located more distally from Linng Gu, in the center of the metacarpus of the index finger and touches the bone.

The next 3 points form a group called the **Three Layer Group**.

For those familiar with Tung acupuncture, these are points **77.05**, **77.06** and **77.07**.

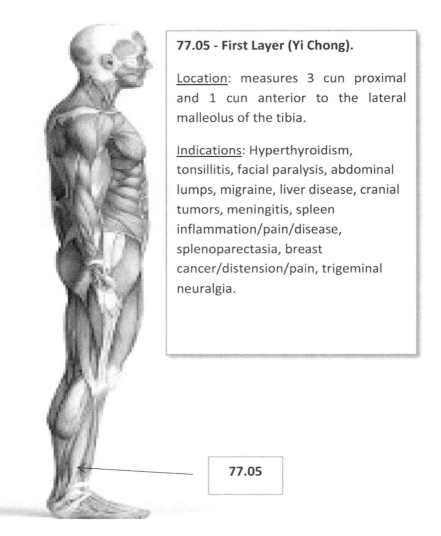

77.05 - First Layer (Yi Chong).

Location: measures 3 cun proximal and 1 cun anterior to the lateral malleolus of the tibia.

Indications: Hyperthyroidism, tonsillitis, facial paralysis, abdominal lumps, migraine, liver disease, cranial tumors, meningitis, spleen inflammation/pain/disease, splenoparectasia, breast cancer/distension/pain, trigeminal neuralgia.

77.05

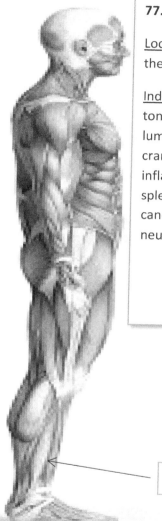

77.06 - Second Layer (Er hong).

Location: Measure 2 cun proximal to the first layer (77.05).

Indications: Hyperthyroidism, tonsillitis, facial paralysis, abdominal lumps, migraine, liver disease, cranial tumors, meningitis, spleen inflammation/pain/disease, splenoparectasia, breast cancer/distension/pain, trigeminal neuralgia.

77.06

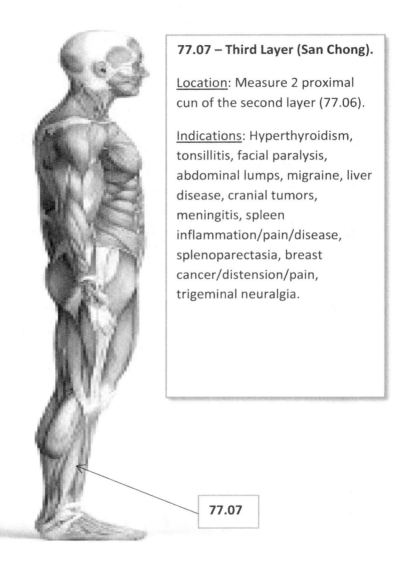

77.07 – Third Layer (San Chong).

Location: Measure 2 proximal cun of the second layer (77.06).

Indications: Hyperthyroidism, tonsillitis, facial paralysis, abdominal lumps, migraine, liver disease, cranial tumors, meningitis, spleen inflammation/pain/disease, splenoparectasia, breast cancer/distension/pain, trigeminal neuralgia.

77.07

Technique for puncturing these 3 points: Insert the needle to a depth of 1 to 2 cun. The first, second and third layers should be used together. They are really effective for the pathologies described. I recommend inserting it in the leg opposite the affected cheek.

The terms distal means away from the head and proximal means towards the head.

It is recommended to look for a point of pain just around the point, if found, it is the point to puncture.

Next we will deal with the fourth point, called the **Central Nine Mile (88,25)**.

Central Nine Mile is also known in Tung acupuncture as the **neuralgia killer**.

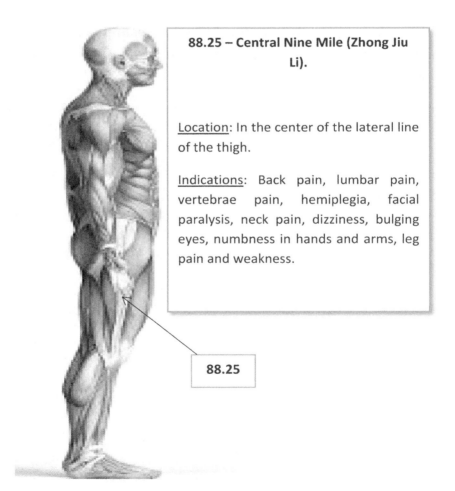

88.25 – Central Nine Mile (Zhong Jiu Li).

Location: In the center of the lateral line of the thigh.

Indications: Back pain, lumbar pain, vertebrae pain, hemiplegia, facial paralysis, neck pain, dizziness, bulging eyes, numbness in hands and arms, leg pain and weakness.

88.25

Puncture technique: Insert the 8 fen needle to a depth of 1.5 cun.

1 fen is about 3.2 mm (depending on the patient). This is one tenth of a cun.

Distal means away from the head and proximal means closer to the head.

It is recommended to look for a pain point just around the point, if it is found, it is the point to puncture.

The last and fifth point is **Seven Miles (A01)**.

Seven Miles is part of Master Tung's Extraordinary Points

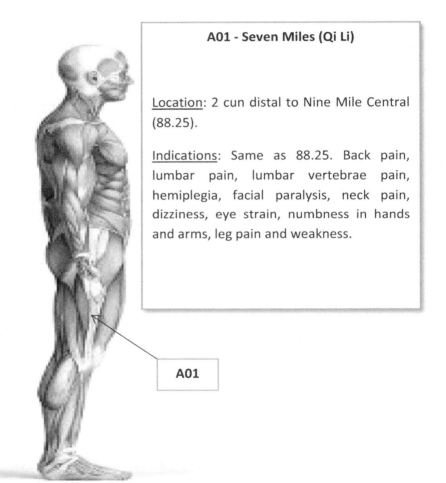

A01 - Seven Miles (Qi Li)

Location: 2 cun distal to Nine Mile Central (88.25).

Indications: Same as 88.25. Back pain, lumbar pain, lumbar vertebrae pain, hemiplegia, facial paralysis, neck pain, dizziness, eye strain, numbness in hands and arms, leg pain and weakness.

A01

Puncture technique: Insert the 8 fen needle at 1.5 cun.

In Tung acupuncture, it is recommended to leave the needles in place for 45 minutes. You can tonify the points by turning the needles clockwise (provides heat) or you can disperse them counterclockwise (provides cold).

The way of being and acting of evolved people consists in cultivating the body by calmness and nourishing life by frugality......
by calmness and nourish life by frugality... Directing the body and nourishing the essence, sleeping and resting in moderation, eating and drinking appropriately, harmonizing the emotions, simplifying activities.
Those who are inwardly attentive to the self, realize all this and are immune to perverse energies.

Wen Tsu Classic (2nd century B.C.)

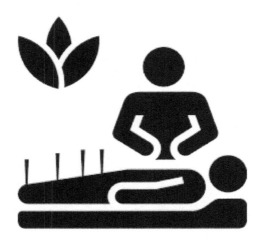

Part of healing is in the willingness to heal.

Séneca

EFT – Tapping

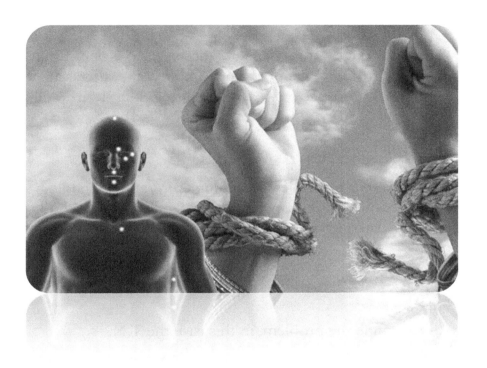

EFT - Tapping (Emotional Freedom Techniques) is an emotional release technique that involves tapping on specific meridian points while repeating phrases related to the issue or problem you are treating.

In this way, a calming response is sent to the body, and the amygdala recognizes it as a safety indicator that helps to calm the nervous system and restore the energy balance in the body.

Physical problems as well as emotional problems (side effects of chronic pain such as stress, depression, phobias, insomnia, T.N. etc...) can be eliminated surprisingly quickly because it rebalances the body's energy system.

With Tapping, the patient receives a scientifically approved tool to support and amplify the therapeutic process during recovery, thus ensuring long-term well-being.

How does it work:

Based on the principles of acupuncture and psychology, finger tapping targets specific nerve endings in the body, while associating specific phrases.

Steps to follow:

1. Determine the problem, in this case the T.N.

2. Measure the emotional intensity of the problem between 0 and 10.

3. Tap on the eight points while speaking aloud or quietly - five to seven taps on each point and sentence.

4. Then measure the emotional intensity of the issue between 0 and 10.

5. As a general rule, it is best to reduce the intensity of the "negative" to 5 out of 10, before moving on to the positive, then continue tapping on the positive until the negative emotional charge has decreased to 3 or less.

Explanation of the points:

KP: The Karate Point (abbreviated as KP) is located in the center of the fleshy part of the edge of the hand (any hand) between the top of the wrist and the base of the little finger, or..... in other words... the part of the hand that you would use to make a karate move.

Cr: Crown. If you draw a line from one ear, through the head, to the other ear, and another line from the nose to the back of your neck, "Cr" is where these two lines intersect.

E: Eyebrow, just above and next to the nose. This point is abbreviated "E" for the beginning of the eyebrow.

SE: On the bone next to the corner of the eye. This point is abbreviated "SE" for side of the eye.

LE: On the bone under the eye, about 1 inch below the pupil. This point is abbreviated "LE" for lower eye.

BN: In the small area between the bottom of the nose and the top of the upper lip. This point is abbreviated "BN" for bottom of the nose.

UL: Halfway between the chin point and the bottom of your lower lip. This point is abbreviated "UL" for under the lips.

Cl: the junction between the sternum (breast bone), the clavicle and the first rib. To locate it, first place your index finger in the U-shaped notch at the top of the sternum (near where a man's tie knot is). From the bottom of the U, move your index finger down toward the belly button for 2 cm, then to the left (or right) for 2 cm. This point is abbreviated "Cl" for clavicle, although it is not on the clavicle itself. It is at the beginning of the clavicle and we call it the clavicle point because it is much easier to say than "the junction where the sternum, clavicle and first rib meet".

UA: On the side of the body, at a point located at the nipple (for men) or in the middle of the bra strap (for women). It is located about 10 cm below the armpit. This point is abbreviated as "UA" under the arm.

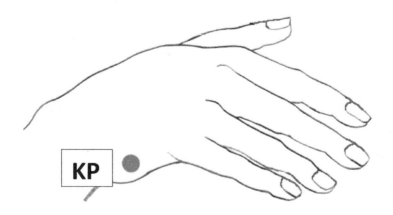

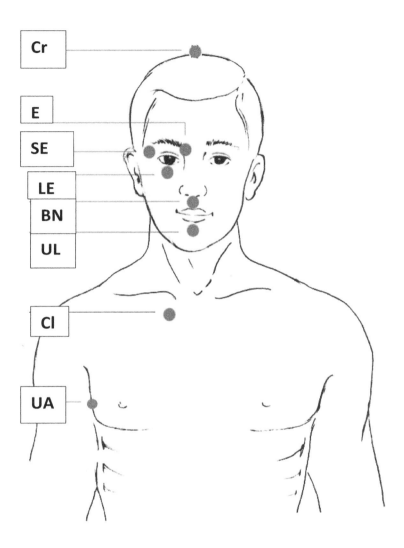

Cr

E

SE

LE

BN

UL

CI

UA

- Some tapping points have two points, one on each side of the body. For example, the "eyebrow" point on the right side of the body has a double point on the left side of the body. You only need to tap one of these two points. However, if you have both hands free, you can certainly tap both sides.

- You can also switch sides when you stimulate these points. For example, you can touch the "karate point" on your left hand and the eyebrow point on the right side of your body. This makes it more comfortable to perform the tapping process.

- Tapping is done with two or more fingers. This allows you to cover a larger area to ensure that your tapping is covering the right spot.

- Although you can tap with the fingers of either hand, most people use their dominant hand. For example, right-handed people tap with the fingers of their right hand, while left-handed people tap with the fingers of their left hand.

- Tap about 5 times on each point. It is not necessary to count the number of taps because any number between 3 and 7 taps on each point is sufficient. The only exception is during the preparation phase when the Karate point is tapped continuously while repeating some standard formulations.

The process is easily memorized. After tapping the Karate Chop point, the other points move down the body. The eyebrow point, for example, is located under the crown. The side of the eye is under the eyebrow point. And so on down the body.

Application of Tapping:

The language we use is always aimed at the negative. This is essential because it is the negative that creates the energy interruptions that are cleared by the basic EFT tapping recipe (and thus brings peace to the system). The EFT method must target the negative in order to neutralize it. This allows our natural positives to come to the surface.

Opening statement

"Despite the fact that I have trigeminal neuralgia,

I accept myself deeply and completely / I choose to let go now / I choose to relax now!

1. **Karate Point**: Even though I have trigeminal neuralgia, I deeply and completely accept myself.

2. **Karate point**: Even though I have trigeminal neuralgia, I choose to let go of this disease.

3. **Karate point**: Although I have trigeminal neuralgia, I choose to let it go now.

4. **Eyebrows**: This pain in my face...

5. Side of the eye: This unbearable pain (throbbing, sharp, terrible, (whatever you prefer))...

6. **Under the eye**: It takes so much joy out of my life...

7. **Under the nose**: Nothing I do really helps...

8. **Chin**: So many things I've already tried to get rid of my pain...

9. **Collarbone**: I am so tired of this pain...

10. **Underarm:** Already so long without success...

11. **Crown of the head:** This trigeminal neuralgia pain is so frustrating.

Take a deep breath and always ask after 2 or 3 cycles: How has the pain changed? How are the numbers now? Have they increased? Have they decreased? What has increased? Has the pain changed?

Then we can proceed to a new positive cycle this time:

Positive cycle:

1. **Eyebrow:** I'm willing to give it another shot.....

2. **Side of eye:** I feel safe enough to let go of all my pain

3. **Under Eye:** I choose to erase this pain in my body...

4. **Under the nose:** I know I can live without pain...

5. **Under the lip:** and free myself from all my pain...

6. **Collarbone:** I choose to relax at this moment...

7. **Under the arm:** and let go of all my tension and pain...

8. **Crown:** All my tensions and pains now dissolve completely...

.

Epilogue

At this point, you have an arsenal of alternative therapies in your backpack to get rid of your trigeminal neuralgia safely and permanently, always under the supervision of your doctor. With only the first three phases, if you follow the step-by-step instructions, you won't need more. If you want to increase the speed of the process, add one or more optional treatments. Some of these treatments do not require specialists and others, like acupuncture, do. You can always use acupuncture points with acupressure or laser therapy to do it yourself, except in the case of zonal acupuncture which requires needles.

I hope you have understood that not all health problems can be solved by drugs and that if we go deeper into the subject, we will realize that, unfortunately, allopathic medicine has changed a lot in the last decades and other darker interests often prevail. I hope that I have taken the blindfold off and that you are now aware that there are other alternatives that go to the very heart of the disease, cutting the root of the problem in a natural way, a way that has been forgotten since the pharmaceutical companies have taken control of the medical market and your health. It is possible that these beliefs, falsely and erroneously installed in your subconscious, are so deeply rooted, that you were not aware that there could be another reality to find that longed-for relief you seek, without going through drugs. It is also possible that you realized that the chemical drugs were damaging you and pulled the band-aid off yourself some time ago. Whatever the reason for your change in perspective, a new horizon has opened up in front of your eyes. Challenging your beliefs is the best thing you can do for your being to begin your healing journey. At the end of this treatment, your life will have changed in many ways, and you will never want to go back. When the eyes see the light for the first time, they never want to go back to the darkness.

We have seen the importance of the involvement of food in the healing process of any disease, regardless of its severity. Indeed, eating is not the same as feeding. It is impossible to heal the body if we do not stop ingesting what makes it sick. In other words, not just any food will do. There are foods that rob you of your health and foods that give you your health. We need to be very clear that not everything is good for maintaining a healthy body and mind. We often hold the false belief that to suppress hunger is to feed ourselves. Just as drinking alcohol or industrial refreshments is unhealthy and cannot replace water or fruit and vegetable juices, so is nutrition. I am always surprised when people ask me about supplements to combat a condition, but none of them ask me the most important question: what am I doing wrong or what should I avoid? My question is, what's the point of wasting your money on supplements if you're feeding your pathology with junk food?

Now that you are free of this blindfold, you have the answers to all your questions and the solution to your problem.

Welcome to your new healthy life…

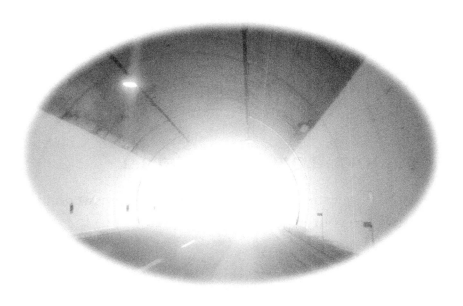

Once the blindfold is removed, nothing is ever the same again …

I remain at your disposal by e-mail:

alqvimiaancestral@gmail.com

FACEBOOK : ALQVIMIA ANCESTRAL

You can ask questions that I will be happy to answer and you can share your experiences with me.

Acknowledgements

To my Life Partner who has been by my side in the best and worst moments. The person who supported me like no one else could and without whom I would not have written this book. I will never be grateful enough to her.

To my little girl, the smile and the engine of my life.

To my Thought Adjuster who never leaves me.

To my readers.

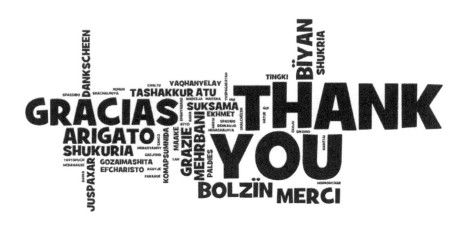

References

Guerrero Alex, How I Defeated trigeminal Neuralgia 2022. Ediciones KDP.

Guerrero Alex, L'Occulte Vérité de l'Hypertension.2022. Ediciones KDP

Moraga Gajardo José Raúl, La Gran Guía Homeopática para la Salud. 2013. Editorial Mandala.

Dr. C. Norman Shealy, Enciclopedia Ilustrada de los Remedios Naturales. 1999. Edición Könemann Verlagsgesellschaft mbH.

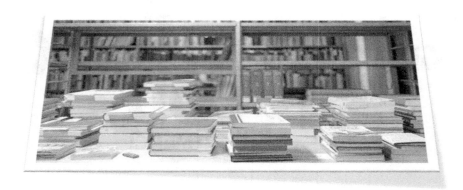

Index

From the same author

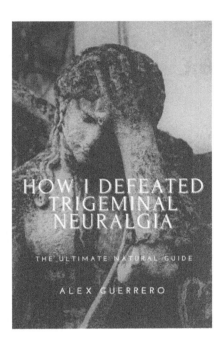

*When you change the way you see things, the
things you see also change.*

Wayne Dyer